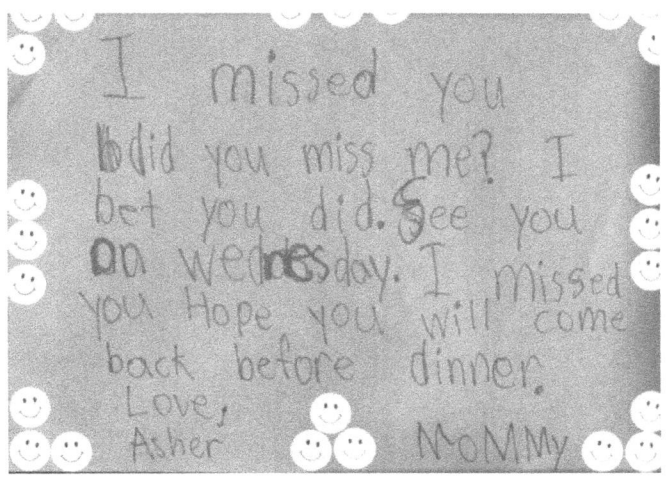

I missed you
Do did you miss me? I
bet you did. See you
on wednesday. I missed
you Hope you will come
back before dinner.
Love,
Asher        MoMMy

I love you mommy. I have
ben praying formyou. I am
exided for you to feel
beter.

"This book has got something important to say and work for God to do in it. Janice is a true Lyme Evangelist!"
**Cindy A.**

"You are AMAZING. I read your book and it's amazing. You're my hero like no joke. I hope that one day, I can be as strong and as inspiring and positive as you."
**Caity B.**

There are so many people in the world that need to hear this hope. It's a story that can encourage and uplift, and not just for people with Lyme, for anyone struggling in chronic illness.
**Rose K.**

"A new day dawning and realization Thank you SOOOOOO MUCH!!!! I am telling you, I can never repay you for your kindness, encouragement and prayers for my daughter."
**Joni B.**

"Living the way you do isn't easy to jump into, but its healthier and I am NOT getting sick again. Thank you for all the information and guidance to living and surviving this thing."
**Jennifer S.**

"All these natural products and methods can sure be confusing, thanks for being someone I can talk to about it and get experience and knowledge from."
**Tamara A.**

How can we "walk in the light," when our journey through life has taken such a horrible detour, such as the many people experience, who are suffering from the extreme life-altering effects of chronic Lyme disease?

The struggle to trust and love God, and to follow His lead in regaining your health, in spite of the symptoms that are affecting the entire body, mind, and spirit, is not just a day-by-day thing with Lyme disease, but a moment-by-moment decision.

Janice Fairbairn's book, "My God, My LYME: Discovering Success in Life Through the Storms of LYME" is a testament to God's faithfulness. Janice poured the very essence of her heart into this book. I am reminded of the lamentations of suffering and the ultimate glorifying of God that King David did in the book of Psalms. Indeed this book is a modern day book of Psalms.

I encourage you to read this book. The hard won lessons that Janice learned in her moment-by-moment physical and spiritual battle are a lifeline for anyone struggling through the many and varied storms that life may bring.

Take the journey with Janice through her discovery of deeper spiritual awareness and truth that lead her to successfully conquering her inner and outer struggles through years of debilitating illness.

**~David A. Jernigan, D.C.**

# My God, My Lyme

## DISCOVERING SUCCESS IN LIFE
## THROUGH THE STORMS OF LYME

JANICE FAIRBAIRN

*For my husband, thank you for bailing water to keep our family from sinking when I was so sick. Thank you for encouraging me to do this project and helping me overcome the difficult obstacles along the way. Thank you for believing in me.*

*For my children, thank you for your precious prayers and countless notes of love and encouragement. Thank you for carrying a load that most kids don't and shouldn't have to emotionally process. May this serve as a memorial for what God can do.*

I remain confident of this:
I will see the goodness of the LORD
in the land of the living.

Wait for the LORD;
be strong and take heart
and wait for the LORD.

(Psalm 27:13-14)

7

# Table of Contents

# Acknowledgements

Thank you for to my Savior who did not abandon me in the Valley of Shadow of Death, and who provided wisdom and stamina to complete this project. It is His testimony of success, not mine.

To my parents and in-laws for the endless support during the darkest days, the hand holding, the praying and the cleaning and research.

To my overnight bunky - Rose Marie, for throwing the football, cleaning my kitchen, for keeping my family together, your loyalty, your friendship, your optimism and laughter.

To Denise M., my Las Vegas surgery chaperone.

To my drivers - Kathy C., Beverly P., Lisha C., Denise M., Kirsten H., Amy R.,Vinny and Teresa G - thank you for delivering me and my kids safely and dependably.

To Mrs. Register - an amazing answer to an unspoken prayer.

To my church family - thank you for the prayers, the endless encouragment and amazing heartfelt support that helped us survive.

To my angel editor- Cindy A., your brain, your verbose vocabulary have enriched my audience, your sacrifice and encouragement and prayers.

To my bible study girls, for the prayers, the help and the support.

To my Jewish angel for the meals and grocery shopping.

Dr. David Jernigan, Dr. Aric Cox, Dr. David Jowdy for listening, blessing and healing - saving my life

Dr. George Watson, who has since joined the angels in heaven, for listening and putting me on the right path toward finding Lyme. May your legacy be far reaching.

To my other angels who changed sheets, picked up my kids, arranged playdates, hired cleaning ladies, text messages of support and encouragement.

# Introduction

This book targets the Lyme patient who feels abandoned, desperate, and alone in this illness. Beyond the physical ravages this illness leaves in its wake, God alone knows your pain, loneliness, agony and discouragement. I want to show you how He can meet you in this dark place with the light of hope.

We all have felt and are feeling your pain quite literally:

- Insomnia for almost a decade coupled with seizures and joint pain that rendered her entire body inoperable

- Entire nervous system felt like it has the constant jitters and tingles

- Hot burning coals are dripping down or being pulled from the brain constantly

- From me, whose chest and throat were constricted, whose nausea was so intense I dropped over 25 lbs to well below 85 lbs

Are you a parent of a Lyme sufferer? Are you a parent suffering through Lyme while trying to raise kids? Maybe you are married to a loved one suffering immensely in Lyme. I pray this book offers you the one thing we all need in this "valley of the shadow of Lyme", a rod and a staff of comfort and hope.

David lamented this phrase in his struggle with sin. Jesus himself from the cross cried out with the same words, "My God, my God, why have you forsaken me? Why are you so far from saving me, so far from the words of my groaning? Oh my God, I cry out by day, but you do not answer, by night and am not silent." (Mark 15:34) The hope God intends for you comes as

13

His grace in this valley, a hope this book attempts to reflect. Be assured, He hears our cry and he answers.

You are not alone. You are not an island left to desolation in this terrible storm. I have felt what you feel; I have met dozens and know there are thousands upon thousands that feel what you feel. The pain, the uncertainty, the desolation, the discouragement, the "no one is listening", and the "no one can fix this" – you have company where you are and where you have been. Most importantly, you have company where you are going, because God is in your tomorrow.

He promises that he will never leave you or forsake you.

# 1

**What in the Lyme is this and how did it get here?**

*The soul knows what to do to heal itself, the challenge is to silence the mind. - Caroline Myss*

Before this chronic illness began, I had incorrectly classified Lyme in with the flu. I defined Lyme as something you could "catch" or "get" and then after a round of antibiotics and a short rest period, you would be back on your feet. Where did this misconception come from? I couldn't have been more wrong. Dead wrong.

Imagine Lex Luther (classic bad guy from the Superman series) has invaded your body; he has drilled into organs, your brain, heart, and liver and set up shop. He has used his cunning "villain powers" to determine if any other bad guys have passed through before and have not completely been evacuated. Any ruffians who have been hiding in dark corners waiting for the opportune moment to strike are found and he alerts them that a strike is indeed eminent and that he has organized it and will be in charge.

Lex Luther is a commanding, in-control villain and he knows how to create the environment in which all like-minded minions will thrive. He pays them well, feeds them well and knows that they will set up shop at his beck and call. You just envisioned the wicked power of Lyme disease as Lex Luther.

Now visualize that Lex Luther is also smart enough to recruit. Before he entered your body, he spent years recruiting other famous bad guys like Mr. Freeze and The Joker to hang out with him so closely that when he entered your body, they came with him. Silently, they lay in wait--poised for the perfect opportunity of weakness when they will launch their stealth approach. Using your own genetics -- a bad heart, early onset para-menopause -- they create a wave of destruction. A scattershot of symptoms becomes their unilateral smokescreen that virtually defies diagnosis. Lex and company are in residence before you know what hit you.

Doctors are baffled and patients are left perplexed. The Lyme continues this approach shifting the front of the war all around rendering the audience confused. Lyme laughs and delights as it takes another victim. Watches as the spiral of symptoms spin both the victim and the doctors into a dizzy state of cluelessness.

Meet Lex Luther under a microscope, your Lyme spirochete medically called borrelia, his wicked partners: babesia and bartonellis. The other ne'er-do-wells? They are usually known as mycoplasma and sometimes also Rocky Mountain Spotted Fever, West Nile Virus and a multitude of parasites. The internal villains? They can be parasites, viruses like Herpes or the flu, bacteria like the common cold. They all join forces and work their collaborative efforts for this commander of the troops.

Let me confess that I am not an expert in Lyme disease, its origination or its life and eradication. What I am an expert in is

16

surviving it. There are many books out there to give you a scientific history and explanation on how this wicked spirochete works. Many are listed in the resource section at the back of this book. When I fell severely ill and found out I had Lyme disease, I could care less how it worked and where it came from. I wanted it gone. I wanted to survive.

I didn't want to hear how effectively it worked and what it could do to my body and why I felt what I did. I didn't want to make eye contact with the bad guy that I was going to assassinate. The Most Wanted in my body just had to be conquered and kicked out.

The most important thing I did learn, however, was that it does not leave quietly. It does not like to be kicked out and because it has been working in stealth slowly organizing over time, it takes layers and time to remove. The leaving of the Lyme was actually harder than the catching it and living with the symptoms that had appeared. The evacuation required stamina, courage and a strength that I didn't possess. It required a supernatural strength that only Jesus could provide.

*Journal entry: I tell you some days I just want to kick this Lyme disease's "a$$" I get such an anger and meanness that wells up inside of me when I watch my kids suffer because I suffer. When I watch mom's suffer because their children suffer from this disease, I want to take up arms and fight against it and destroy it. It is in these moments that I begin to recite things like "in Him we are more than conquerors". Okay God then let me conquer it and be more than this disease.*

*I lay in my detox bath and I cast it out. I have been speaking to my body and to the disease, asking it in no uncertain terms to vacate. I am speaking to the Holy Spirit himself indwelt in me and CASTING IT OUT. Thanking God in advance for already working. Today, as I prayed and wept, I pictured myself as the woman who reached out to just touch the edge of His robe because she knew that simple act would heal. I believe and I recognize that the Holy Spirit lives in me. This indwelling, which is even more powerful than touching cloth as the robe of Jesus, and just by that one touch she was healed instantly. I pray that the Holy Spirit will use that same power, and similar to a light switch, heal me entirely.*

*"If anyone says to the mountain go throw yourself in the sea, and does not doubt in his heart but believes that what he says will happen, it will be done for him. Therefore, I tell you whatever you ask for in prayer, believe that you have received it and it will be yours." Mark 11:23*

*Lord I pray that you rid me of all unbelief from this flesh and mind and renew my heart to your promises that my belief may remain strong and steadfast. I have been saying to his mountain of Lyme – go to the sea, go to the sea, go to the sea. I will not ask nicely, I will not plead; I will just command and YELL – GO TO THE SEA.*

*You oh God, to you be the glory and praise for its departure and my complete healing and that of my children.*

A full frontal battle against Lyme disease becomes a 5 alarm fire, all hands on deck – flank them from every direction. The battle plan involves multiple doctors, a willing insurance company, family members, friends, a church community, money, patience, time, energy and a spiritual strength that is only supernatural. The warning label should read: Do not try this stunt at home on your own.

# 2

## How in the Lyme did you get in here?

*To name a thing, in other words, is to bless God for it and in it.*
*Ann Voscamp*

I had no ground zero bull's eye rash or bite that I remember. Over 50 percent of Lyme patients don't either. My stealth season grew slowly through increased weird skin reactions, diminishing tolerance to foods that I could eat, a miscarriage, early Para-menopause, chest pain, shortness of breath, angry days and other uncontrolled emotions. All were most likely over a period of 10 or more years, maybe longer.

After my symptomatic explosion and first ER visit 10 years into this, I did receive a positive on a blood test for Lyme – surprisingly. Most do not. The IgenX lab test is the most reliable, but unless your immune system has launched a counter attack, then it will go undetected. Now please, do not take that to mean that you should launch an attack. Some say, take antibiotics for a few weeks, take some herbals (i.e. Cat's Claw), to set things in motion to prompt the immune system to react and therefore get a positive on the test. I have to ask you why? Why would you cause yourself undue pain and suffering. The ammonia and neurotoxin release cannot be "controlled" and you have no idea how much will be dumped onto your system and how strong your system is to handle it.

19

Why do you feel you must have the positive on the Lyme test to begin treatment? Do your symptoms register on the list? Are there any other mysterious illnesses that could explain what is going on with you? There are forms of testing available that are non-invasive and do not require this blood test. Muscle strength, kinesiology or bio-resonance testing are incredibly reliable to detect Lyme and all its components. (See the resource page for more Information).

I was unknowingly testing my immune system. I had been taking Cat's Claw for my high cholesterol in quite high doses. Dangerous if you have Lyme. That is what actually caused the crash and, to God's glory, that I did not perish from it, but He used it to guide me.

When I received my positive on a Lyme test, it was an answer to prayer. I never thought I could say that knowing I had something so terrible could be an answer to prayer, but it was. It had a name. Ann Voscamp describes a similar experience in her book "1000 Gifts" where, through her husband's research, they thought they found what she had been struggling with. They both felt relief as well, from the finding, and from identifying the enemy. She says "when you don't have a name for something, you're haunted by shadows, it ages you." She goes on to say:

"Now, in the Bible a name.....reveals the very essence of a thing, or rather its essence as God's gift....To name a thing is to manifest the meaning and value God gave it, to know it is coming from God and to know its place and function within the cosmos created by God. To name a thing, in other words, is to bless God for it and in it."

How is it possible to name this thing, put a target on its back to destroy it and thank God for it at the very same moment?

Trying to chase the causing of my angry and tired days, a naturopath doctor attempted to balance my hormones, stimulate my adrenal glands and lower my cholesterol simultaneously. Oh, you want a symptoms list? Early symptoms were the hormones and flat out adrenal failure/crashes. Also, I had been registering very high eye pressure with my eye doctor for over five years with no glaucoma anywhere in the family and no high blood pressure. Though a recent cholesterol test came back elevated, I countered with exercise and eating. We had been eating organic, gluten free, dairy free for years. My body struggled – in what should have been my healthiest season of my life – and I wanted to know why.

The "perfect storm" in my body exploded from a combination of stress, some of the "natural" remedies and supplements, para-menapause, older pregnancies, and some genetics. Those supplements actually started killing the Lyme and my "crash" that happened was actually one big crazy giant herx explosion.

Understanding a "herx" will help you recognize it and give you the ability to name it on this journey. A herxheimer reaction is defined as a bacterial sepsis – which means a toxic dump on your body that puts it into shock. You know when you jam all the potato peels down the drain and have a momentary slowing and backing up - that is your body's immune system in a herx.

For Lyme sufferers, though, the bad news is that Lex Luther, upon his death, planned in advance and has set deadly traps to explode in order to exact posthumous havoc upon you when he exits. He releases deadly neurotoxins into your bloodstream. Those neurotoxins flood the body's systems and cause a "sepsis" in all the filtering organs – the liver, kidneys, and bowels and invade the brain causing what we call "brain fog".

By comparison, the venom of a poisonous snake bite contains neurotoxins. That tiny amount in the bite of snake venom has the power to paralyze and kill within hours. Lead poisoning and the destructive effect of tetanus are all similarly an attack of neurotoxins.

That crash, or giant herx explosion, began a series of events in my body that set the stage for all the Lex Luther invaders to have a party. A party that flooded my system with enough neurotoxins to give me brain fog, hindered vision, and vertigo and began to start shutting down my filtering organs one by one.

Questions blare into your conscious thought like "where did I get this?" and "how did it take over?" Let's address the noise and move on. It's pointless to focus on it.

A wise doctor asked me in turn, how does a tornado form? You have to understand that in Kansas, this question is so appropriate. Well, a tornado forms because the conditions have to be just right. Pressure, moisture, fronts – all have to be in synchronicity and in the perfect setup for a tornado not only to form, but to have power and destroy. The same is true of how and why Lyme disease explodes; the conditions have to be right. Genetics, eating habits, stress, physical weaknesses, exercise, pregnancy, etc. can all be part of the "conditions" that are formed to allow Lyme to get a foothold.

If faced with Lyme, the conditions in your body were there, whether we like to face it or not and most of those conditions are likely out of our control. Stop berating yourself and trying to solve the "ground zero" question. That question cannot be answered – not today and maybe not ever. "How am I going to conquer this illness?" becomes your new focus. Shift all your mind's attention to beating this thing. The past is the past and your future lays wide open. We've named it, looked it in the eye and wondered where it came from. Now, where do we go from here?

Finding a qualified doctor or Lyme treatment program addresses the most important thing you can do as a Lyme patient. Make sure the doctor listens and if he tries to put you on antidepressants, run for the door. If he can help you get rid of the neurotoxins in your brain, then you won't need antidepressants – tell him you will happily dance a jig instead. Believe in your symptoms, do your research, pray and find that doctor or team of doctors who believe in you and believe in healing. If the doctor knows about herxing, neurotoxins, detoxing the body, and Post Lyme Syndrome, then you have found a good place.

*Journal entry:*

Am I going blind? My new level of acceptance is praying that this is not to be my plight in this illness, but that His will be done. I continue to feel like my vision is failing me, the eyes are not acting right, I can't focus to read anymore. I struggle to read the devotional with the kids in the morning and my Bible in my quiet time. Everything is not necessarily blurry, although at times I experience double vision, it is more like that it just hurts to look at things, hurts to focus at all and my mind just cannot decipher the words on a page. The worst times are going into a big store like Lowes or Target or going to church – looking at something farther away, in bright lights. I squint but my legs still go weak and I feel like I am going to throw up or pass out.

I literally haven't been to church in months because I cannot stand to look at anything in the church without getting physically ill and weak. I tried again to go to church for Christmas Eve thinking I was doing better and spent the whole service sitting staring at my lap or looking at the lady's sweater right in front of me to prevent further nausea.

Why Lord would you prevent me from corporate worship when I need it most? As a trained painter, the artist in me screams in desperation about losing my eyes. Losing the ability to see the world of color and beauty, and on top of that I love to read. Completely love to read. Losing that ability in this illness has been beyond devastating. I have so much time on my hands to just lie and I can't sleep and can't read.

The wonderful thing you Lord have helped me discover in these times is how much more time I have to spend with you. When I get caught in the grip of a "fear" like this going blind one, I have to pray scripture then start vigorously praying for others. It's the only way my focus will turn from me and back to you and rid this fear.

In the vacuum of chronic Lyme, try not to focus on yourself. Self-focus only exacerbates the pain and agony, loneliness and pity party. Don't spin your wheels wondering, use all your energy to live and survive. When you are left to your own thoughts, take them captive and redirect your attention on praying for others. The mind shift from your load to others' needs eases the burden and gives rise to a healthy prayer life.

# 3

## To Name a Thing

*Start by doing what is necessary, then what is possible, and
suddenly you are doing the impossible.*
*St. Francis of Assisi*

Getting discouraged creates a commonplace event during this valley. Sitting in front of doctor after doctor who won't listen and can't help feeds the hopelessness. Take heart, because I have yet to meet a Lymie who hasn't run through the gamut of doctors – I think the highest count is 42. Yep, a sweet little 14 year-old girl who had been to 42 doctors who could do nothing and had done nothing to help her, until I met her at the same clinic where they actually heal Lyme.

Being around other Lyme patients on the journey can be the light you need in the storm. Other people who know it can be beat that will cry and pray with you through your deepest part of the valley. My husband and parents and friends all loved on me and prayed for me, but they don't know what it felt like and what and how I struggled. But my doctor (a former Lymie himself) and the patients I met turned into a lifeline. Their gift to me: a ray of hope in this present darkness. This monster would not get the best of me.

It was 3 months into my treatment for Lyme and I was doing better, recovering, eating, and putting on weight. I went with a girlfriend to Wal-Mart to buy Easter stuff for our kids. Now at this point in my life, I didn't go anywhere alone. I still wasn't driving; my eyes were still terrible, no reading, no driving, and no church. I barely had the energy and strength to walk in to the store from the parking lot – probably weighing in still way less than 95 lbs at 5'4".

I was also a mother, who wanted to bring some joy into the house after all the devastation. My kids needed normal – they needed a mom who could fill Easter eggs and hide them. They needed something in their world to be predictable and normal. So off we went to Wal-Mart that day.

Well, we did get through a few aisles before the nausea wave hit hard. The weakness in my legs and body hit with such a vengeance, the cart was my only hope of remaining standing. We quickly made it to the registers, paid and got to the car.

Functioning as a mother still seemed nearly impossible. My household barely held together by the help of family and friends. I felt I was constantly drowning by the lists of things to do and what hadn't been done and all I wanted to do was get better. It was about this time in my treatment that I got hit with a truth: my kids have Lyme too.

Since their births, both of my kids have struggled with many health issues. My son displayed constipation, night terrors, behavior problems, food allergies and eventually Asperger's. My daughter experienced constipation, stomach pain, constant coughing and ear problems, food allergies, sleep problems, emotional upsets, and energy and leg pain. We didn't battle these

28

like normal people, accepting their fate. I tend to be a bull in a china shop and charge through not accepting our misfortune. So we had gone on specialized diets, seen natural doctors and had been "duct taped" together and functioning for about 3 years. That barely held together existence included a rigorously strict diet that included GFCFSF (Gluten Free Casein Free Soy Free) and many specialized--he can eat potatoes, she can eat almonds, he can eat cashews, she can eat sweet potatoes--for each and every meal and 27 supplements given throughout the day just right.

As I lived through this Lyme, learned and lived through the healing of it, I met some other people on the journey, in particular a mother and her son with Asperger's, both with Lyme. She led me to a website about the link between Lyme and Autism. You are kidding me. (The lightbulb goes on above head and I pick my jaw off the ground). Of course, the neurotoxins and ammonia are damaging the neurotransmitters, the brain, the Autonomic Nervous System (ANS). All things that Autistic Spectrum Disorder (ASD) kids struggle with could be caused by neurotoxins and ammonia poisoning. Why aren't doctors testing for Lyme then in autistic kids? Urgggh. More frustration with the lack of knowledge of this disease.

Also, there is very little research about how Lyme can be transmitted or if it can be sexually transmitted or en utero. Well, I did my own little test. I took my kids in and had them tested and they had every single little critter I had – the trifecta of Lyme (borellia, bebesia and bartonellis), Rocky Mountain

Spotted Fever, West Nile Virus, mycoplasma, parasites. Everything. So, science theory proved out in my house, yes Lyme disease can be passed en utero. As for the sexually transmitted, my husband was tested and did not have any of them. Unsure that is conclusive enough, but it lends more credibility than the scientific reports I have read.

So, while still undergoing treatment myself, we began treatment for the kids. Now, they were not chronically ill like me, they had not had an explosion. The conditions in their bodies were not ripe for an attack, their youth and our healthy lifestyle with all the supplements were keeping it at bay so we knew we had to go in immedieately and get it. Clearly, we now understood why we had been living life "on eggshells" for their entire lives.

Remember, I could not hold my own life together yet. I still couldn't drive, couldn't read, couldn't go grocery shopping. Now, I had to manage and advocate treatment of killing this beast of Lyme out of my kid's bodies too. The nightmares of herxing were still very raw. I agonized over going after this Lyme in there little weak bodies. I wouldn't wish a herx reaction on my worst enemy, let alone my own children. I had to trust this method of treatment would keep their herxing at bay like it had in mine. But how on earth would I have the mental capacity to do appointment and treatments for them on top of mine?

Years ago I took flight lessons in a Cessna 172. One particular instructor was a young guy and in our first lesson he did his best to impress me. Heart failure began when he held my

30

hands back and pushed the plane up at a steep angle (to me it seemed straight up). I could be exaggerating, my husband accuses me of that all the time, and I was too busy freaking out to read the dials. For the sake of drama let's just imagine it was a steep ascent, shockingly steep. The instructor proceeds to let go of the yoke while holding back my hands and says "watch this." Ummmm, really?

As humans we are built to avoid disaster, not watch it. Well, maybe watch someone else's disaster, but not our own without some sort of reaction. But as I sat there panicking and fighting the urge to grab that yoke or punch that guy (oh, you have to know he was so fired after we touched down), an amazing thing began to happen. The plane's nose began to sharply dive and correct itself. Then, it corrected again back up, then back down less steeply. Each time it rose and fell until it had leveled itself out for flight. The plane is built to know where "flying normal" is.

God made our physical bodies this way. As much as we despise pain, pain tells the body something is wrong and it needs to be corrected. At times, the body just needs a little "help" and it will eventually self-correct. That is what I love about the doctors who treated me for Lyme. They are in the business of helping the body self-correct. With proper support, detoxification, nutrition and exercise, the body will sustain itself at its "normal" flying pattern. It is also amazingly able to adhere and adjust to a fuel system built on junk food and laziness and drugs. But that flight can only last so long.

31

I'm telling you this, Lyme patient, because just like in the plane lesson, those steep corrections on the way to leveling out did not seem to me to be a normal flying pattern. The plane knew where it was going and how to get itself there. But remember, those initials corrections had me holding my breath. That is how this "healing from Lyme journey" can be for your human body.

The body wants to self-correct and has been trying to eradicate this beast all on its own, but the neurotoxins clog up the systems and they can't work as intended. Unclogged and supported, the systems and the body will get rid of the Lyme. Along this journey of corrections, though, there will be white knuckling that can cause you to think you are going to crash and you will want to bail. Ride it out on the down, wait for the up and the down again.

Many times I wanted out, I wanted a quick fix; I wanted a drug to put a stop to how I felt. God kept reminding me that I was fearfully and wonderfully made (Psalm 139) and through the help of the doctors who got me well, I knew that God's plan for how my body should heal superseded any quick fix or temporary plan.

There is a song by Chris Rice called "Teach Us to Count the Days" that I have been reminded of lately since my perspective of all things busy has been shifted to all things in neutral and in limbo. I took for granted my health and my planning until the valley hit. The chorus of the song says "teach us to count the days, teach us to make the days count, lead us in better ways, that somehow our souls forgot, life means so much, life means so much." But my favorite two parts are for today, "will I compose a curse or a blessing" and that "every day is a bank account and time is our currency."

How am I going to spend my time, being a blessing to others and myself or just buried in the busyness of life? Don't get me wrong, there is still laundry to do and cooking and errands and kids sports practice, but do I handle it all as if it's a blessing now or do I curse the busyness and grumble and flush those minutes and that currency?

In this valley, this struggle, don't miss the opportunity for God to revamp your spiritual outlook on life and reboot your soul while your physical body balances back out. Get out of His way, let Him get at the heart of the matter. It's why He has brought you here in the first place. Character always trumps comfort as an agenda item for our Lord with regard to our souls.

I was re-reading the 23rd Psalm and it occurred to me that the valley of the shadow of death is sandwiched between such goodness in this passage. Before I walk through the valley of the shadow of death (which before Lyme, I had no idea how it felt or what this phrase really implicated), He makes me lie down in green pastures. So He ensures I have had sufficient rest and rejuvenation before He leads me to the valley. He leads beside still waters and restores my soul, so He shows me his beauty and peace reminding me of His awesome creation and power and strength before the valley. Then He leads me. I didn't accidently end up there, He leads me to the valley, which means He is there with me.

Then will I walk through the valley by His side with trust as the rod. The staff removes the fear because I focus on the things He is doing for me and has done for me. While I am in the valley of the shadow of death, He is preparing a table before me for me and my enemies. I don't know about you, but if I'm having a party and I am inviting my enemies, it must be quite a shindig. (which is a really really big party, for those of you are don't speak southeast Missouri hick talk). And what is He going to do at this feast after my valley? He will anoint my head with oil and overflow my cup so that goodness and mercy will follow me all the days of my life and I will dwell in the house of the Lord forever.

I could not live through the valley of the shadow of death without knowing this truth of the Lord's presence with me.

It was everything.

It was the deal breaker.

In my lowest of lows, the truth of His presence beside me satiated the longing for health and the emptiness of pain and sorrow. These promises are so rich to claim and know that for every valley, there is a mountaintop and his goodness and mercy will follow me all the days of this life until I get to dwell in His house forever.

### *Journal entry:*

*Sitting in the dark on an airplane, flying to see a doctor who can hopefully fix the problem of blood clogging in my brain, I begin to physically fight symptoms that catapult my body into an all-out mental and spiritual battle as well. Do the people I see know how I feel? Did they see me get wheeled on to the plane on a wheelchair and wonder what a not quite 40 year old is doing so thin and so sick and frail? Do the people see how I feel, how much pain and fear? My heart begins its dance of arrhythmia and palpating and the uneven throbbing creeps up the left side of my neck and starts to beat uncontrollably through my temple and back down to my heart as if it could explode any moment. Simultaneously, my throat tightens as if someone is trying to choke the very breath from me and I feel as if I can't swallow. I begin my deep breathing and prayer to bite through the episode, not knowing if this is the one that will be short at 30 min or long at 3 – 4 hours. I feel as if my entire insides are trembling and tingling and my feet feel like an electric skillet has them captive on high heat.*

*Then I hear it in my ear and my soul at the same time "Because he lives, I can face tomorrow, because he lives, all fear is gone. Because I know, I know he holds the future; life is worth the living just because he lives."*

*Ok, there it is, He is in my tomorrow, with or without the surgery and the pain. Praying for comfort, praying for rest, praying for the Holy Spirit to take control of my physical body and weld it back as the Creator himself intended. I am flying to Las Vegas to have surgery on my CCSVI to repair the blood flow drainage problem the Lyme created that is causing all this trouble. I pray I actually survive the trip to make it to the surgery and fight the urge not to imagine what havoc is created if I go into cardiac arrest or stop breathing right here on this plane. When you physical body is in such a crisis, taking those thoughts captive for Christ is an all-out WAR on which you have to live on the front lines full time.*

*Then I hear again, "Seek first the kingdom of God and his righteousness, and all these things will be given to you." (Matthew 6:33)*

*Why this verse God, Why this message in this pain crisis on this plane ride to surgery? Is it that simple that it all boils down to my priorities? I want to feel better and heal and to raise my children and serve my husband, hasn't that been driving my fears all along? God, if I'm healed, wants me to serve Him first and glorify His kingdom first. Not my will or my plans, but yours.*

*Wasn't I just last week on a good day, thinking about normal life resuming and making plans? MY plans, mind you, not His.*

*"For His thoughts are not my thoughts, nor are His ways my ways." Isaiah 55:8-9*

*I always read through the Old Testament and thought what a dreadful stubborn and stupid people those chosen Hebrews were to forsake the blessing and forget His faithfulness. Oh, how I completely understand now. When I'm blessed with strength and healing from Him alone, what do I do now with that time and energy, give it to Him? Or start to go my own way again and make my own plans? How many bouts with the rough patches and regressions is it going to take before the pattern is set correctly toward His favor?*

*In the book the "Land Between", the author, Jeff Manion says in the valley is where our habits are made. The Israelites had quite a habit of whining and ungratefulness in their valleys. Is that the habit I want to make in this vale? Or one of complete reliance and trust on my Maker?*

*As I look out the window of the plane at the mountains we are flying over I hear one more verse from my Lord resound in my heart "I look my eyes up to the hills where does my help come from. My help comes from the Lord, the maker of heaven and earth." (Psalm 121:1)*

For those of you Lymies that have been living in the panic cloud of sheer pain, this book is designed for you. My heart breaks for all the people who are living this and have no hope. After completing this book, I pray that you find newfound hope and ideas for how to survive your storm of Lyme. Join my community on Facebook www.facebook.com/justlivinglikethiswithLYME or with me on Pintrest http://pinterest.com/jpfairbairn/just-living-like-this-with-lyme/ or on Twitter https://twitter.com/janicewithlyme. Get connected and stay in touch.

# 4

## Suffering in Lyme

*I thank you, o Lord, for all the suffering you send me. I beg you to send me a 100 times more if you think it is right. I shall rejoice if it pleases you to afflict me without sparing me in any way, for the accomplishment of your holy will is my greatest consolation.*
St. Francis of Assisi

One of the greatest gifts God offered me through this illness was a better "suffering index". Lyme and its sufferings surrounded me like a cloud. Stifled and claustrophobic, I found fear in that suffering. Suffering filled my panic cloud. One night, God chose to shift my perspective. In the middle of a terrible night that I that I thought would be the death of me, He began to bring people to mind to pray for. I would be praying and begging for myself and then He would bring someone to mind to pray for. The time passed more quickly and with less anxiousness on my part. The pain never left, but the fear did.

Praying for others in my suffering became an amazing gift that was not on the horizon. What a great example of God's omniscient inclusiveness. God recognized I needed to know that I was not alone in a valley, I was not the first and I would not be the last. Without caring for these people fighting their own fights, I would have completely fallen victim to the biggest pity party on earth. Knowing this about myself, at times I still threw small congratulatory celebrations for my issues. But then, as I

38

would focus on what I didn't have, God would press into mind people's needs again. Could I imagine walking in their valley?

- Putting my one month old into surgery to save her from a kidney disease that could or could not save her life?
- Having my 35 year-old husband fight one of the worst, most aggressive types of cancer on the planet?
- Watching my 9-year old go through treatment for an inoperable brain tumor and still die?
- Have my husband abandon me penniless and leave me for a someone that was considered a friend?

Now, let's go to the biblical suffering examples God gives us in His word. "I have suffered much, preserve my life, Lord, according to your word." Psalm 119:107 The psalmist holds fast to the idea that God is our anchor in this life's storms. He knew regardless of our acceptance of the valley, it is ours. There exists no other way through it than to depend on God to navigate us and keep us afloat. He ends this phrase with 'according to your word', because he is going to hold fast to God's promises.

I tried to imagine while in my valley what would it have been like to have been anointed to be king. And like David, in front of God and everyone I knew at such a young age (1 Samuel 16:13). Then give Goliath to defeat in front of the king, his brothers and the whole army (1 Samuel 17). David was a national hero and a child prodigy. If you read the tabloids today, you know what happens to child prodigies in our culture. They get inflated egos, too much too fast. All the money and attention burns them out. The pressure to be great is huge, the limelight too bright and they quickly fall to drugs or alcohol to cope. David had a lot to live up to, but he also had in his pocket a lot of God's promises for his life.

For added unwanted pressure, King Saul begins to get jealous and tries to kill David, not once but twice and then sends the army in pursuit of David. Could I imagine being on the run from all the safety and security I know? Could I imagine spending my time in the valley wondering if I had done something to have God remove his favor from my life but yet still believe? Could I handle this valley all alone?

David's psalms have been such a comfort to me. He shows his heartfelt anguish and fear and yet his anchor held fast. He never held back his feelings from God himself. This lesson serves us well today. Tell God your heart in the valley. He knows your suffering; give it to him. The psalmist says in Psalm verse 116, "Sustain me, my God, according to your promise, and I will live; do not let me hope be dashed." Ask God for hope to sustain you in your valley.

There can be a lot of "deal making" that happens in our minds and prayers from the valley floor. We've seen examples of it in many Hollywood movies, but in our hearts, we know that we are thinking we can offer something, anything that will change this course or save us. We humanly think somehow we can reason our way out of the pit like we can a speeding ticket.

David reminds us who holds absolute power, in verse 19, "but who is like you God?" He is God, needing nothing from me, leaving me no power to negotiate to get what I want. But yet, we have examples of the petitions of saints in the Bible "changing" God's mind. Didn't Abraham negotiate over the cities of Sodom and Gomorrah? Don't our prayer and petitions make a difference? Oh, yes, our prayers, petitions and questions are necessary to be in relationship with Him. Petitions yes, but deal making no.

Believing David again from his valley cried out in anguish and then praised. In Psalm 71, he talks about giving his testimony and he reminds God in verse 18, "Even when I am old and gray, do not forsake me, my God, till I declare your power to the next generation, your mighty acts for all who are to come." One of my fabulous go-to books in the past 2 years has been 31 Days of Praise (see resource list). It taught me how to praise in my anguish. Pain and praise go hand in hand in God's native tongue.

David promises to praise Him, to tell others of His faithfulness. David says "Though you have made me see troubles, many and bitter, you will restore my life again; from the depths of the earth, you will again bring me up, you will increase my honor and comfort me once more." (Psalm 71:20) "Sacrifice thank offerings to God, fulfill your vows to the Most High, and call on me in the day of trouble; I will deliver you and you will honor me." (Psalm 50:14-15) David believed and had a track record with God acknowledging faithfulness does have benefits.

The Lord met me and spoke such gentleness to me through my suffering. Allow your heart to be open to the dialog of

41

getting to know Him and how He can provide relief. God reminds us in Isaiah 49:23 that "Those who hope in me will not be disappointed."

The benefit will look different to all of us. For Job, "God blesses the latter part of his life more than the first" (Job 42:12) and Job "died old and full of years." (Job 42:16). For David, his benefit took the form of being honored and leaving a legacy through collecting the money to rebuild the temple through Solomon.

One of my heart-friends and mentors would frequently quote the book of Job to me in my valley and encourage me to read it. I couldn't. I just couldn't make eye contact with more suffering. Job lived as the person God shows us in the Bible who suffered the most. Layer after layer of suffering and I couldn't look at it in the eye, couldn't study it. Why? Because I think deep down I knew this valley of mine could get deeper, could get worse. I wanted to traverse it right where it was, not a step lower. I mean, I couldn't even handle it where it was, how could I handle more tragedy, more suffering? I possess quite a vivid imagination and to fight off the other cloud in my life, the fear cloud, I couldn't give my mind any more ammunition for the enemy.

Call it what you will, but denial coupled with fear leads to isolation. I hid from things that fanned the flames of my fear. I ran from people or Bible stories that implied more suffering and increased my panic cloud.

When I lived in New York, my sister and I used to joke about the traffic. Sometimes we would sit through a huge traffic jam and there wouldn't be any construction, any wreck, and no bad weather. My sister coined this phenomenon "traffic for traffic's sake". But, in a typical situation where an actual car wreck existed, the traffic jam would be due to "rubbernecking" as you go by. Something in us must make eye contact with someone else's tragedy or misfortune. We feel forced to slow and look, no matter how tragic, right?

But I will tell you that in a valley in the middle of my own misfortune, I didn't want to look any tragedy right in the eye, not even my own. Head down like I'm was headed straight into a rainstorm, just trying to get past it. When I prayed for others in my suffering cloud, I refused to imagine any worse. I couldn't imagine any worse; I couldn't make eye contact with it.

The apostle Paul managed to confront his aversion tendencies, "That is why I am suffering as I am, yet I am not ashamed, because I know whom I have believed and am convinced that he is able to guard what I have entrusted to him for that day." (2 Timothy 1:12) I have to believe that God is able to guard my sorrow and guard me and my life that day, this day and the next day, each day through the walk.

Yes, I eventually read the book of Job, once I could keep my head above water. As much as Job suffered, God had put the fence up for how much he would suffer, how much he would let the enemy put upon him in the test. He guarded Job. Proof that God establishes the limits of our suffering.

Trust this truth as you suffer and live through this trial. God has decided how much and for how long. Guarding your life and your edge, He will not let it surpass His purpose and His plan. "The Lord Almighty has sworn, surely as I have planned, so it will be, and as I have purposed, so it will happen." (Isaiah 14:24)

***Journal Entry:***

*A few weeks I felt so much stronger, eating great and feeling like I could even start some yoga and then a ginormous crash again. It has been every few days now that I crash and crash and can't seem to find my footing again. That is the one thing that anyone with a chronic disease will tell you. Once you have had a good day again, once you have tasted the savory morsel of healing, it is complete and utter torture to be returned into another pit. It should provide such hope that you can get there again, but it just dangles there to increase your madness and the inconsistency of the journey makes me feel even worse.*

*I feel like a greyhound chasing that fake bone around the track never to catch it and let it fill my hunger and satiate my desires.*

*"The Lord gives and the Lord takes away. Blessed be the name of the Lord and may His name be praised." Job 1:21*

*I haven't even been able to read the book of Job because I can't look at his suffering and here is this verse in my mind. My self-destructive thoughts cannot handle waiting for the possibility that the other shoe could drop but then God gives me this word from Job. Blessed be the Lord and may his name be praised. Can I praise him from my valley?*

*A devotional I read the other day reminded me that it is better to be in darkness with the Lord than in the light alone. I know that truth and my heart knows that truth, but my mind in this illness has a terrible time falling in line with everything else. Does my doubt come from my mind alone or does it come from my heart? Do I have enough promises and truth written there on my heart that I am sure that I will make it through this?*

*"I am confident of this. That I will see the goodness of the Lord in the land of the living. Wait for the Lord, be strong and take heart, and wait for the Lord." Psalm 27: 13-14*

*I get so overwhelmed by this promise when he whispers it back to me. I really will make it through this and it will be for a good reason. "All things work together for the good of those who love him who have been called according to his purpose" Romans 8:28*

*Taking every thought captive for Christ has never been so hard and I am a recovering addict. In addiction, he completely removed my desire. In Lyme, he has not removed the pain or the suffering. It's almost like I had to be so weak and humbled by this illness and its situations, that when I finally relinquished control of it to God, then the Holy Spirit took over the wheel of my heart and is directing it and all the traffic around it! It is He that is in me that will guard my heart and mind in Christ Jesus.*

*And if I want the Holy Spirit to drive, the more "gas" I put into my heart, the more God can use it to direct and speak to me. And what if I am so saturated in goodness that the tank is full for God to use all the time? Oh that I knew more scripture by heart, so to keep the dialog going and keep hearing his voice speaking to me whispering promises and telling me what I need to hear to keep on keepin' on. Then he surprises me by using other things from my past like old hymns. I never thought that all those many verses of Alberta on the organ in my Methodist Church would help me in this valley but they have resonated in my soul.*

*Great is thy faithfulness, O God my Father, there is no shadow of turning with thee. Thou changest not, thy compassions, they fail not. As thou has been, thou forever will be. Great is thy faithfulness, great is thy faithfulness, morning by morning new mercies I see. All I have needed, thy hand has provided. Great is thy faithfulness, Lord unto me.*

*I never knew that in my upbringing in a traditional church that all these songs were so branded on my heart and those decades later, He could use them. It became quite clear to me that every ounce and minute of my day needed to be drenched in truth. Christian music of all kinds plays in the background at home and in the car – verses taped to mirrors and windows. Everywhere I look there is something that even my subconscious can sink into my heart to be used to "hear" God's voice whenever the Holy Spirit wants to speak to me.*

Hope buffers suffering. At the end of the valley (because there will be an end), we will not be disappointed. Our God will memorialize and set apart something in our testimony for the suffering. He just does, faithfully. "May the God of all hope fill you with all joy and peace as you trust in Him, so that you man overflow with hope by the power of the Holy Spirit." Romans 15:13 "Those who know your name will trust in you, for you the Lord have never forsaken those who seek you." Psalm 9:10 "Be joyful in hope, patient in affliction, and faithful in prayer." Romans 12:12

Remember, David, said in Psalm 23 that God leads us to the valley and that means he walks through it with us, now picture him guarding you and protecting you in the valley. Just as he did for Job.

# 5

## How Much is Too Much?

*Afflictions are often the black fold in which God doth set the jewels of His children's graces, to make them shine the better. To be left unmolested by Satan is no evidence of blessing.*
*C.H. Spurgeon*

Horatio Spafford and his wife were prominent and successful in 1860's Chicago. They were supporters and close friends of D.L. Moody. He lost his only son to scarlet fever and merely a year later he lost all his business investments in the Chicago Fire.

Aware of the stress of these events, the family planned to go to Europe and join Moody in one of his evangelistic campaigns. Business delayed him, so he sent his wife and four daughters on ahead of him. Nine days later, the ship collided and sank in a mere 12 minutes. He received a telegram from his wife that merely read "Saved alone."

Spafford boarded a ship to join his wife. The captain called him to the bridge to announce the very place they were crossing was the location of the shipwreck.

He then went below deck and wrote the following hymn:

*When peace, like a river, attendeth my way,*
*When sorrows like sea billows roll;*
*Whatever my lot, Thou has taught me to say,*
*It is well, it is well, with my soul.*

Could there be any story closer to the story of Job? How much more suffering could this one man take? A sweet lady from my church community brought over the box set of Selah worship hymns during my trial, since I couldn't read much, music was such salve to my soul. I tear up even still to hear their version of his song.

*It is well with my soul. Though Satan should buffet, though trials should come, let this blest assurance control, that Christ has regarded my helpless estate, and hath shed his own blood for my soul.*

From his valley, Spafford chose to focus on what Christ had done for him and to give thanks. Oh, giving thanks in the trial took the focus off his loss and put it on his gain. Isn't that where our focus should be? Read the last chapter of the Bible, the book of Revelation, and see how it ends.

*The trump shall resound and the Lord himself shall descend and it will be well with my soul.*

King Hezikiah can relate to chronic and sudden illness in Isaiah 38. It states in verse one that "In those days, Hezekiah became ill and was at the point of death." So it was quick, it was sudden and it took him straight into the valley of the shadow of death. Not only that, but the Lord told him in the same verse to "Put your house in order because you are going to die, you will not recover." Now watch for the amazing thing. Instead of discouragement from the king, we see hope and confidence mixed into his tears of sadness. He says, "Remember how I have walked before you faithfully and with wholehearted devotion and have done what is good in your eyes." Then he weeps bitterly, sadly.

How comforting for other sufferers to know that Hezekiah also wept, and wept bitterly. He held such sadness and loss of this life so suddenly; his devotion, his good work for the Lord, his family, his legacy. The king is leveraging any hope for an end of suffering on his personal devotion to God.

But watch as the Lord responds to him in verse 4, "Go and tell Hezekiah, I have heard your prayer and seen your tears and I will add fifteen years to your life". Here displayed God's awesome response, and His promises continue "And I will deliver you and this city from the hand of the king of Assyria and I will defend this city." So fifteen years added to his life, the protection of his city, AND fighting off a mortal enemy and still the Lord has one more thing to say. "This is the Lord's sign that the Lord will do what he has promised. I will make the shadow cast by the sun go back the ten steps it has gone down on the stairway of Ahaz."

Why so much more? If you look back at what Hezekiah said in verse 3, he didn't even actually ask not to die. Implied in his sadness, wishing quietly not to die and most likely God read it in his heart. So without actually asking, but rather an indirect request to not die, God gives him 15 years, protects the city, defeats his enemy and seals it with a supernatural sign.

God loves signs. Throughout the bible we see him display something physical to help us spiritually. Noah, Moses, Joshua, Elijah, the list goes on and on. He longs to covenant with us and mark it, memorialize it, seal it. It's the dot on the "i" to how he finishes his promises – more like an explanation point. And what does this seal - all this extra blessing - do for Hezekiah's faith? Keep reading starting at verse 10 and see the heart of a king, a man who knows his maker and trusts completely. My favorite part begins at verse 17, when Hezekiah says "Surely it was for my benefit that I suffered such anguish. In your love you kept me from the pit of destruction; you have put all my sins behind your back."

Surely it is for your benefit, Lymie, that you are suffering such anguish and physical ailment. Think about it, if this suffering has no good purpose, how could a person ever endure it? How could anyone possibly live another minute holding on to this physical life, if no good can come in the course of suffering, not just at the end of it?

Hezekiah finishes by saying "For the grave cannot praise you, death cannot sing your praise; those who go down to the pit cannot hope for your faithfulness. The living, the living – they praise you, as I am doing today; parents tell their children about your faithfulness. The Lord will save me, and we will sing with stringed instruments all the days of our lives in the temple of the Lord."

If death would have taken me quickly from this disease, would I have the opportunity to share of the Lord's good work and his faithfulness? I can praise the Lord from heaven, but the one thing I cannot do in heaven is tell of his faithfulness. I cannot witness, I cannot testify from heaven. Suffering is the time clock of active testimony.

"By the blood of the lamb and the word of our testimony" we will overcome (Revelation 12:11). We will overcome the enemy by Christ's death on the cross AND our testimony. It is a weapon I have in my arsenal to use here and only here on this little blue planet.

My son's teacher gave me a book called 31 Days of Praise and it is almost as tattered as my Bbible now. Those devotions have been gone through over and over and over. The cycle will not stop. I will praise Him in the valley, in the suffering because it is for my benefit to focus upward and build a testimony for His kingdom. Praise is the best focus shifter there is. Praising kept me from a pity party. Praising Him in the suffering shifted my focus above the clouds, out of the valley entirely, and into eternity.

### *Journal Entry:*

*Ugghhh, as I stop off the scale fully clothed and not hitting even 90 lbs. holding my purse. God, please don't have me melt away. I know I can't get well unless I am strong, help my body to eat and gain weight.*

*These are the prayers I utter so often as I watch myself wither away. I was not a big person to begin with and so my small frame could not afford to lose 5 lbs. let alone the over 25 it has lost.*

*This morning I was reading in Luke 12 and this part of the verse jumped out at me "Do not worry about your life, what you will eat, or about your body....."*

*Before that passage always meant not to worry about where your next meal was coming from, but now I realized it applied to my situation as well. He, the God of the universe knit my body together, he was its creator and he would be its physician healer. Trust him, let him guide me and stop*

51

*worrying about the weight, how much I wasn't able to eat and how frail I had become. He still had me in the palm of his hand.*

*It goes on in verse 29 to say "Do not set your heart on what you will eat or drink, do not worry about it." Let it not be my main focus in healing, but to be on him and things eternal. I find that now I have a completely different understanding of the shackles of my flesh. I have battled my flesh in addiction, but to battle my flesh in disrepair and continue to temper my spirit on things above, remains a battle still.*

*I have taken for granted this earthly vessel, this gift of life, until now. This body has always responded and one what I needed it to do. To have this vessel fail, I finally long for my heavenly body – the one that will never fail, that feels no pain or brokenness. The bodily form that is more like God's – perfect in form and never houses sadness, despair or discouragement. I yearn for my new vessel and see how my view of the flesh on earth has shifted.*

Trust in this promise from God during the dark days. The days when it seems your physical vessel has separated from your very soul and won't accept nourishment, medicine, treatment or liquids. God created you and He will tend to your every need, physical and spiritual.

*Here I am! I stand at the door and knock. If anyone hears my voice and opens the door, I will come in and eat with that person, and they with me. (Rev 3:20)*

# 6

## Tears in a Bottle

*I don't need easy, I just need possible.*
*Bethany Hamilton – Soul Surfer*

I don't need permission to cry; in fact I come from a long line of criers. Ask my mom, ask my sisters, and especially our better halves. From a commercial, to a testimony, to a tired - hungry -long day, we like to and can cry easily. I thought I might run out of tears in this illness and turned around a generation of crying for my daughter, but alas, I cannot run out of tears.

Emotional tears differ so much from these tears of sadness, deep mourning, savage fear, loss, uncertainty and anguish. In these Lyme tears, this illness had me pinned down and sapped out. I told my husband it was not my lack of emotional control or spiritual strength, it just feels like a 300 lb. giant gorilla sat down on my panic button and wouldn't leave. I was red-lined and cried often.

I came across these verse after reading a book or devotional (and for the life of me I can't remember which one – one of the many consequences of the brain fog – I forgot everything), "Record my misery; list my tears on your scroll – are they not in your record?" (Psalm 56:8)

Did that pierce your heart dear Lymie and bring more of these precious tears to your eyes? He, the Creator of the

53

universe, the Lord of heaven and earth, lists my tears on His scroll, your tears.

They are recorded, every single one.

Every single one.

And not just the tears, but the misery, the sadness, and the ache that goes along with them. The Message translated it like this: "You've kept track of my every toss and turn through the sleepless nights, each tear entered in your ledger, each ache written in your book."

Oh, how I needed to hear that he tracks and knows my toss and turn, my sleepless nights, every ache of my heart with these tears. My favorite version however comes from the New King James Version "You number my wanderings; put my tears into your bottle."

In my Lyme brain fog, I needed to know that he numbered my meandering, my lost-ness, and my fog along with catching my tears in His bottle. Just picture that for a moment. A room with shelves in heaven lined with ache and tears all logged in His book. He says "For you, Lord, have delivered me from death, my eyes from tears, and my feet from stumbling, that I may walk before the Lord in the land of the living." (Psalm 116:8)

When he delivers us from death's grip forever and we arrive in heaven God promises that He Himself will "Wipe away every tear from their eyes" (Revelation 7:17 ). "He will swallow up death forever and The Sovereign Lord will wipe away the tears from all faces." (Isaiah 25:8) Maybe each of us gets to smash open our tear-filled jars in heaven to celebrate that there will be

54

no more! Heaven is the cease-fire zone for crying, an anti-pity party!

As we leave our biblical examples of suffering, we have to rest on one more place: Calvary. I couldn't make eye contact with Job, but could I with Christ and his suffering? Could I have survived that prayer session in the Garden of Gethsemane alone if I had known the future and acknowledged what I had to face ahead? Could I have handled the past 18 months of suffering if I had known what was coming would be the actual valley of the shadow of death?

I think that I would have been like Jonah high-tailing it out of there on a boat to Tarshish with Nineveh in my rearview mirror, saying "whewww, that was a close one." But not our Lord Jesus. I couldn't make contact with Job's suffering, how could I even bear to look at my Savior's agony at the cross?

Maybe it was because Jesus is both human and God. Or maybe because I knew His death and resurrection so well. Perhaps in knowing how He suffered for me, it helped me carry this burden for just one person, not all of mankind. Jesus had such a purpose for his sacrifice and suffering and He had that awareness going in. I have absolutely no idea why this illness came into my life and what the Lord will do with it.

He walked into the valley of the shadow of death knowing where he was going and did it willingly. He did it alone. He did it completely alone.

This part is almost the most unbearable for me. I had an incredible community of people praying and supporting me. His best friends stopped praying and started sleeping. Not the kind of prayer warriors you'd bring to your most important fight ever. That behavior belonged more on like the B team prayer warriors – falling asleep. He did it alone. The book of Isaiah says in chapter 53:3 "He was despised and rejected by men, a man of sorrows, and familiar with suffering."

Oh, He knows your suffering and He didn't just walk through the valley of the shadow of death. He walked to it and took the keys of Hades right from the owner. "Surely he took up our infirmities and carried our sorrows....He was pierced for our transgressions and crushed for our iniquities." But it ends by reminding us "and by his wounds we are healed." (Isaiah 53:3)

The writer of Hebrews also says in chapter 7:25 "Therefore He is able to save completely those who come to God through Him because He always lives to intercede for them." He not only suffered more than any of us can fathom, He did in willingly, obediently, sacrificially and most important, COMPLETELY. He lived to die for us, He lives still to intercede for us. When you are afraid and in the darkest place in the valley remember:

"That God is down in front. He is in the tomorrows; it is tomorrow that fills men with dread. God is there already. All the tomorrows of our life have to pass Him before they get to us. The savior has tried for himself all the experiences through which he asks you to pass; and he would not ask you to pass through them unless he was sure that they were not too difficult for your feet or too trying for your strength." – Streams in the Desert (F.B.M.)

***Journal Entry:***

*Everlasting, your light will shine when all else fails, never ending your glory goes beyond all fame and the cry of my heart is to bring you praise, from the inside out Lord my soul cries out. (Hillsong United)*

*As we were worshipping this morning in church, this song wrenched in to the deepest depths of my heart. The "cry of my heart" takes on a whole new meaning. I am reminded of the verse in Proverbs 2:3 that we can call out for insight but also cry aloud for understanding. I have often wondered if I would run out of tears and that God would tire of my anguish and exhaustion. I have reached the bottom of myself and actually get disgusted with how weak and helpless I feel. Crying seems to be the only emotion I have left. Where is the spectrum of emotion the Lord created for us to enjoy and pass through the seasons? Have I only one temperature setting of late, only one feeling to feel, is there no other lens to look through, not other antennae getting a signal?*

*I remember growing up in the country, how frustrating and hilarious if was to try to tune in a TV channel on the antennae. We had to do a balancing act on our heads like playing Twister – contorting to get in the station and stay there because it worked better if you held that spot.*

*I feel so limited, so closed off when the wave of anguish covers me and engulfs me in tears. Drowning in sorrow is a feeling I had never known and to feel it in the very depth of my soul, my heart and my complete physical self is beyond my own coping mechanism.*

*My mind and heart are thankful and grateful, but my soul grows weary at swimming in grief and sadness, my eyes grow tired of crying. I want to pick up the self-pity and cast it instead into this giant pool of tears so I can swim somewhere else. Where is the pool of contentment and joy, where do the streams of peace flow? Where is the waterfall*

57

*of hope that I can dash these frustrations and self-focus over the top so they can crash on the rocks of salvation and strength and disappear into the pool of eternity?*

*My life is in you Lord, my hope is in you Lord, my strength is in you Lord, in you, in you. (Daniel Gardner)*

*I am not alone on this journey, because You Lord have carried me, you have sustained me, and you have healed me. Your faithfulness has spoken to me through your saints, through their prayers, through their cards and through your servants. Thank you that you have never forsaken me and the pool I swim in you have placed me in, not to drown in sorrow, but to cling to you my raft, my boat, my Savior. Lord help me ride in these seas trusting you as my Captain. You know the way and you provide peace wherever I am.*

Just picture it with me – God has a special place in heaven for your tears. That is the only thought I want you to contemplate as we continue this journey. In your darkest places and the deepest quicksands of depressions through Lyme, remember to imagine your shimmering bottles of tears. I wonder if they become iridescent when God's glory shines through them?

# 7

## The Valley of the Shadow of Death

*Live by his promises, not by explanations. Expect the mystery of*
*God's providence.*
*- Dr. Adrian Rodgers*

I had a very vivid dream one night in the first few months of this illness. I was some sort of spy detective soldier person on a stakeout after some bad guys with my fellow team members. I got shot, but it luckily hit my bullet proof vest. They radioed in for help and kept telling me I was not going to die but would make it. As they were loading me in the ambulance, I distinctly remember telling one of my partners, "I can't die yet; Lance (my husband) doesn't know how to give the kids their supplements."

Even in my subconscious thoughts I was wrestling how my husband and kids would survive in my absence. At that time, before we knew the kids had Lyme, we had been on a 4-year journey trying to duct tape together their health. Just like holding the antennae at just the right angle on one foot to get that TV signal, if we gave the kids supplements each day in the right amount and combination (27 total between the two of them) and the correct foods (they were both allergic to different ones) then we could get through the day and to the next one. Being the mastermind of this process, I researched went to doctors and created the plan, memorized the plan and executed the plan.

The only people we could leave the kids with overnight were my parents, because my dad, as a nutritionist and scientist, could follow my three pages of instructions. There was masking tape on shelves in the pantry, the kitchen, sharpie marker written on food boxes – all instructions to keep the flow going correctly in the house. I was terrified that if I died, the kids would go to ruin because no one would be able to keep them duct-taped together in this system. So paranoid for my poor husband to have to do this upon my departure, that I called over a girlfriend and made her copies of the plan and educated her on the system just in case.

Tell me, dear Lymie, what extreme plans and dire thoughts have you been having and wrestling with in this valley? Some are in denial and others are drawing up wills. Such a difficult place to be: to make plans and to not dwell on them. When they say to prepare for a rainy day, they need to remind you not to do it in monsoon season.

I get it. For months, it genuinely surprised me that I woke up the next morning. On the days with the inability to sleep, shocked that morning ever came. I stood at death's door for about three months. For months after that I lived in the yo-yo of relief and despair, back and forth. I first wrestled with being there at all, too young, so suddenly, but soon the "why" portion of the struggle ended and I landed somewhere different.

- I had work left to finish – like raising my children
- I had unfinished business that had before gone unnoticed – the regrets of the undone

- I felt trapped between planning and unplanning

"How to live fully in each day but plan to live toward tomorrow. I get it. I get to live. How do we live fully so we are fully ready to die?" (Ann Voscamp in 1000 Gifts). It was here on this precipice of living fully but being fully ready to die that God had me. God placed me here to reconcile many things in my heart and to strip away all things not eternal. This forced me to focus on Him and His plans for my life.

Sure, I had unfinished business, but did I have unfinished business for the Lord or was it mine? I, I, I, me, me, me – The more I wrestled, the more self-focused I became. The more I prepared to be ready to die, the more it became obvious to me that my undone list was my own. My purpose in life needed to be refocused on things that mattered long after I was gone.

Do you want to live fully Lymie so you are fully ready to die? How do you balance this act of living fully and preparing fully? The juxtaposition frightens and overwhelms me.

A song by Steven Curtis Chapman echoes in my mind. "I'm living the next five minutes like they are my last 5 minutes, cause I know the next five minutes may be all I have. Every morning God gives is precious, every heartbeat, every breath I take. I'll never have them back once they've left us."

But how do I truly live out that concept? Does that mean no planning, no actual discipline, not washing dishes - how do you plan to not plan? A heart of gratefulness isn't the most difficult part to achieve; marrying this to the reality of the disease becomes the quagmire I find myself in more often. Do I correct the bad behavior between siblings at breakfast? Do I plan to go on a school field trip? Do I plan to paint the kitchen cabinets, or rearrange the furniture? Do I plan a summer vacation not knowing how I will feel?

How do I prepare to die and live fully each day?

### *Journal Entry:*

*At a museum in London, there was a special showing of the work of Edward Munch, famous for his painting the Scream that is a cultural icon. I didn't know much about his work or life before entering. He was a very troubled artist evidenced on the walls as I walked through the show. I could see Munch's anguish build in his work. They had journal entries of his life placed on the wall along with the paintings as a timeline. Toward the end of his terrible life journey filled with tragedy and angst, I find myself standing in front of the infamous 'Scream'. Next to it was a journal entry that I now know by heart.*

*"Over the blue and black fjords, hung blood and tongues of fire and a loud unending scream was piercing nature."*

*I had seen this iconic painting in culture and in art class, but as I stood in front of it, I heard it for the first time. I heard that cry from his soul in anguish. It was terrible, terrific and empty.*

*Is it any wonder that the human condition could survive anguish, physical or emotional or both without Christ? I felt that anguish; I have felt that unending scream pierce my own soul. I never fully comprehended David's words in Psalm 23 of "the valley of the shadow of death." But let me tell you there is an unending scream in that valley of the shadow of death. An unending scream that resonates through every cell in the body and bounces and echoes off the walls of the soul.*

*The valley of the shadow of death was where I walked, where my steps have trodden. I always thought that once I felt God calling me home, I would be at peace and that because I knew my eternal destination, I would have no fear of death. Was I wrong? Why didn't I find peace and comfort in the heaven that awaited me? I don't know if it was because the timing felt so premature, or if I just felt unfinished work on earth, or missing my loved ones. But every cell in my body battled standing in death's door. I had many talks with God there and why I was at that point and how long I would be there. Finally, when the pain and anguish got so great that I reached the point of surrendering and begging for heaven. I thought I was resolved and would go, then He quietly told me 'no'. I was staying but I would stand where I was. The suffering was not over yet.*

*That is why David says a shadow accompanies death – it's a dark cloud, a panic cloud which is difficult to breath in, difficult to talk in, difficult to find a coherent thought in, impossible to see a way out or imagine making it another minute in.*

*I had asked and begged to stay and complete the work he gave me to do here on this earth, and now I had my answer. He granted my request but at such a high price that I wasn't sure I could pay it and complete the task. I was standing at death's door and told I couldn't pass through but had to stand there indefinitely. All I knew is that he knew the number of my days; he knew this illness wouldn't kill me, and then He had to know how I would survive the rest.*

The ebb and flow moments of triumph and despair seem endless in the Lyme battle. Take heart that there is always an ebb and a flow. There is always an explosion and a recovery. It took your body years to get that sick, unbeknownst to you, so give it time to climb out of the hole slowly and then be stronger than ever. No need to scream – at least not unending.

# 8

## Control is an Illusion

*Never be afraid to trust an unknown future to a known God.*
*Corrie ten Boom*

One summer after my freshman year of college, in my first apartment with a friend, we got the cable hooked up and received free HBO for one month. We watched Days of Thunder with Tom Cruise twice every day for months –no exaggeration. It was at the pinnacle of "hotness" in his career, and we swooned. Nevertheless, it turned out beyond hilarious to me that God used a line from this movie one day to get my attention. Cole (Tom Cruise) sustains an accident on the racetrack and becomes scared to race again. His doctor, now his new girlfriend, calls him on it. "Control is an illusion, you infantile egomaniac. Nobody knows what's gonna happen next: not on a freeway, not in an airplane, not inside our own bodies and certainly not on a racetrack with 40 other infantile egomaniacs." See, even cute guys couldn't plan for accidents – life altering accidents.

I am an admitted control freak. Type A, workaholic, persistent to be in control of everything. This year, God ripped that out of my white- knuckled grip and quoted Days of Thunder to me in my frustration over the loss of this control. He knew how destitute, trapped and lost I was. For the first time, I didn't know what would happen next. God answered me with "control is an illusion, you infantile egomaniac". Control most certainly is an illusion. What I thought I was controlling before, I was not. My healthy body existed as a gift from God, not under my control because I ate right and exercised. It was not by my hand that I experienced good health and and it is not by my hand that I am not. I was never in control of anything; I just had to learn that I wasn't.

Lyme disease didn't simply have me feeling at a loss of control though. Lyme had me scared out of my mind. Fear had me grappling in the shadow of death. Fear over who would help my husband raise our kids and if they would do a good job. Who would make sure they knew how to tie their shoes, knew how to protect them, help them make friends and teach them good judgment, knew how to comfort each of their many tears, knew how to show them surrender, true control surrender – how to die to self and love the Lord?

But control does not exist, not here on earth by me. The Creator of the universe, however, is in control. Ann Voscamp says it best from 1000 Gifts "And it is only when our lives are truly emptied that we're surprised by how truly full our lives were. The fullness of joy is discovered only in the emptying of our will." Lyme disease emptied me to the bottom of my well.

The loss of control, the complete surrender changed everything. The curtain torn down, the rookie magician fired and the truth revealed. I had let God into some places, let Him handle the big stuff at times when life came to a crossroad, but I had controlled all the rest. I had not surrendered all of it. Not let Him have the little stuff, the plans, the stuff I could "handle." I robbed God of the credit for the daily bread and the daily breath.

*"Now listen you who say, 'Today or tomorrow we will go to this or that city, spend a year there, carry on business and make money. Why you do not even know what will happen tomorrow. What is your life? You are a mist that appears for a little while and then vanishes. Instead you ought to say, if it is the Lord's will, we will live and do this or that.'" (James 4:13)*

I resolved to live within the boundary of His will. I resolved to make plans within the fences He lays up for my life. At the heart of my surrender came my need to plan.

I have made plans, a lot of plans. I am a plan-maker. At this point, I hesitated to begin, but I was ready to live again, prepared to look forward longer than one minute. My kids needed it, my family needed it, and I needed it. More importantly, God challenged me with life continued – but it would be on His terms. Now, when I make plans, my prayer became that He will allow or not allow them to take place and I will be okay with that.

Some plans worked out, while other feel by the wayside. I did get my kitchen cabinets painted with a friend's help. I didn't make it home to see my sister and my nieces last summer. Disappointment mitigates that hurt, but I am able to negotiate it because it was the Lord's will. He closes doors that could be too much for me. I have limitations now. I live with a realization that I cannot do it all. This new arrangement is from the Lord and I trust Him. That trust in Him brings the peace to handle it no matter what.

In light of that thought, I must remember that I am "one breath away from eternity", as Louie Giglio said so profoundly. My best advice is this: make plans; look forward, but live in the now. Don't live in tomorrow's plans, live in today and make plans for tomorrow. Bathe those plans in prayer and let God shut and open doors as He see fit.

I love when the heroes of the Bible are given to us in their human frailties to allow us to see they are flesh and blood just like us, grappling in their souls. "For to me, to live is Christ and to die is gain. If I am to go on living in the body, this will mean fruitful labor for me. Yet what shall I choose? I do not know! I am torn between the two: I desire to depart and be with Christ, which is better by far; but it is more necessary for you that I remain in the body." (Philippians 1:20-24) Can you feel the tug-of-war in Paul's spirit?

I have been familiar with the verse 21 for years – "for to me to live is Christ to die is gain." That statement alone doesn't get to the heart. That is a head truth. Of course, I know that living here is to glorify His kingdom and to get to be in heaven –that is, to die is a blessing. But as you continue to read these verses, you see his struggle. He's torn between the work to do on earth and to depart to be with Christ. Now remember, Paul met Christ. Jesus transformed his life – from spiritually blind to seeing. He touched, loved and learned from the Master, Raboni, Messiah. He rubbed shoulders with Jesus, the Resurrected Messiah.

I would have thought that would make it a done deal. Just take me there, put me back by Christ's side, and get me to heaven. But Paul clearly says he is torn. His love for Jesus is so strong that the desire to breathe and finish his work on earth puts him at odds in his soul. Just like me. Just like you. But his work was not done.

### *Journal Entry:*

*He said this thing wouldn't take me and yet he holds me here on the precipice of life also with no healing, no forward movement and sometimes with regression I feel I am falling off it again.*

*Job 12:10 In his hand is the life of every creature, and the breath of all mankind.*

*Job 12:22 He reveals the deep things of darkness and brings utter darkness into the light.*

*I asked my counselor yesterday about this grappling with death thing that has kept me in conflict about my faith and eternal yearnings. Why wasn't I at peace at facing death? What was driving my reluctance, my fear of leaving so suddenly, so seemingly undone here? Why, if eternity has been placed in our hearts, in standing in the doorway of death, wasn't I ready to be with our Lord and Savior?*

*My counselor's answer was simple, and I don't know how I missed it. God planted eternity in our hearts, yes. But he also planted the human need to have breath on this earth and to do our work here. To be with family, to raise children, to share Christ with others. There is nowhere else in the space time continuum of heaven and earth that these things can be achieved. "We are God's workmanship, created in Christ Jesus to do works, that He prepared in advance for us to do." Eph 2:10*

*He breathes life into all things. Deut 32:39 "I put to death and I bring to life, I have wounded and I will heal." He gives breath, and until He takes it, we fight to keep it for the continuance of our souls.*

*We know in our most inmost beings that we cannot leave here without permission. It is He who gives and takes away. We cannot yearn not to breathe; it is against the DNA of our creator that we were made in the image of. He planted eternity in our hearts to give us that hope when we are discouraged, when this world gets too hard and we long for something better, to be released. What a beautiful dichotomy He knew we would need. To have the hope of heaven so we don't give up and to have the hope of life so we will fight to keep it and let it be blessed.*

If Paul struggled with the "regrets of the undone", with the work he was put here to do, then so can I. Then so can you. More than all else, hold tightly to the life you have been given. It is a gift from God. It is worth fighting for.

Find your balance between the today and the tomorrow of life. Hopefully being emptied of life has you living more in today that you ever did before. Just don't let Lyme scare you out of planning for your tomorrows. Accept the gift of life and the fight God placed inside each of our souls to keep it.

# 9

## Death is Done

*...Only you can decide how your fires will affect you. Will you be sanctified or scarred?*
*- Beth Moore*

It occurs to me as I have typed it over and over again so far, that Lyme is the shadow of death. Not death itself. But the valley of the shadow of death. Just as we are under the covering God's wing, in the shadow of his protection. Why? Why did he hide Moses in the cleft of the rock? Because the very presence of God himself would be too much for our earthly bodies. Too much holiness, too much glory - so he protects us and only gives us a shadow.

The same remains true of death for the believer. We don't have to experience death. David purposely doesn't say "I walked in the valley of death", but the "valley of the shadow of death." Because that is all the power death has over us - a mere shadow.

Imagine being a prize fighting boxer and only having to experience the shadow of your opponent instead of the actual sting of his punches. Because that is all the power death has over us. We don't have to feel the punch or the sting or the agony of the hits.

*How priceless is your unfailing love, O God! People take refuge in the shadow of your wings. They feast on the abundance of your house; you give them drink from your river of delights.*

*For with you is the fountain of life; in your light we see light. (Psalm 36:7-9)*

Please, hear this! Death has no power over us. Christ lives in me the hope of glory, the fountain of life. We will feast on the abundance. I will never, never have to walk in the valley of death because Christ did it for me on the cross. The only chance death has to scare me is to throw its shadow over me and loom there toward crisis as an empty threat. This valley of the shadow of death cannot grow worse from a spiritual standpoint. That is the bottom; that is the end of it. The shadow is all we will feel. End of the story. Christ walked through this valley, kept going and took all the pain of death for all mankind so we would not have to walk any farther.

Christ walks through it still.....with me, with you. And Christ does not fear the shadow. Walking through the valley with him means we can do it without fear.

*"To shine on those living in darkness and in the shadow of death, to guide our feet into the path of peace." (Luke 1:79)*

*"My body also will rest secure because you will not abandon me to the realm of the dead." (Psalm 16: 9)*

The boundary has been laid, the line drawn in the sand. You don't have to take another step from here. He paid it forward for you. Death's door is closed, not open for business. Imagine that prize fight again - you standing in the opponent's shadow but not feeling a single punch. At the end of the match, the winner is declared and it is you. It is you? The one who didn't take a punch, who only stood in the shadow? Who would fight and win this for you? Christ would. He did. He raises your arm in victory.

*"Therefore he is able to save completely those who come to God through him." (Hebrews 7:25)*

*"So whether we live or die, we belong to the Lord. For this very reason, Christ died and returned to life so that he might be the Lord of both the dead and the living." (Romans 14:8)*

David says in Psalm 18:4-5 "The cords of death entangled me, the torrents of destruction overwhelmed me. The cord of the grave coiled around me, the snares of death confronted me." But then he says of God in verse 28-29 "You, O Lord, keep my lamp burning; my God turns my darkness into light. With your help I can advance against a troop; with my God I can scale a wall." David recognizes the strength of living in the light and so can you.

Because Christ conquered death, all we have to experience is this shadow. This doesn't mean downplay how bad the valley is. The shadow stands vicious and mean. As David said, the pain and agony of it entangle. It is horrible; it is horrific. But Christ has saved us from the worst. He has saved us from its vilest and most awful desolate parts.

We don't know about death because we don't have to. Death is done for the believer. Christ conquered death. Death is done; it's had its day. Let's put a contemporary slant on this.

For any of you Seinfeld fans I picture the Soup Nazi standing at death's door. Instead of sending people away saying "no soup for you", he is sending believers in Christ away saying "no death for you."

Not today. No death for you.

Death is done.

*Then will the eyes of the blind be opened*
*    and the ears of the deaf unstopped.*
*Then will the lame leap like a deer,*
*    and the mute tongue shout for joy.*
*Water will gush forth in the wilderness*
*    and streams in the desert.*
*  The burning sand will become a pool,*
*    the thirsty ground bubbling springs.*
*In the haunts where jackals once lay,*
*    grass and reeds and papyrus will grow.*
*  And a highway will be there;*
*    it will be called the Way of Holiness;*
*    it will be for those who walk on that Way.*
*The unclean will not journey on it;*
*    wicked fools will not go about on it.*
*  No lion will be there,*
*    nor any ravenous beast;*
*    they will not be found there.*
*But only the redeemed will walk there,*
*    and those the Lord has rescued will return.*
*They will enter Zion with singing;*
*    everlasting joy will crown their heads.*
*Gladness and joy will overtake them,*
*    and sorrow and sighing will flee away.*
*Isaiah 35:3-10*

*Journal Entry:*

*Today I wrestle again with death and life. With the maker who gives breath and takes away. My dear friend, my heart friend suddenly departed at 50 years young leaving her 7 year old son and husband in shock. All of us in shock. She oozed Jesus. She lived every minute for Him. The Holy Spirit emanated from her like a beacon and for her testimony on this earth, hundreds were drawn to it in her and came to know Him.*

*Did she not have so much more to offer than me for your kingdom? Here I stand at death's door awaiting a verdict and she was swept through it without so much as a pause or a knowing. Just gone. One heartbeat away.*

*Am I still here because I was doing a bad job? What do I need to do differently if you let me stay?*

*How can I live like Sheryl, whose eyes constantly sparkled the light of Christ, whose laughter resonated? Sheryl, the prayer warrior, who you used to answer prayers for my healing. Sheryl who the last time I saw her said so excitedly "I see it, I see it in your eyes, you are coming back. Hallelujah, you are coming back."*

*Christ responds to me "in this world you will have trouble, but take heart, I have overcome the world." (John 16:33)*

*There is that phrase again. Take heart. Reminding me it is about searing His promises on my heart that my actions and words may reflect them fully. This isn't just a statement of fact or a timeline of events but a promise, a guarantee, a pledge, a betrothal, a commitment. And unfortunately, the first part of the promise is that we will have trouble. All of us, me, Sheryl, her husband, her son. There is no such thing as a trouble free life – what we see on the outside that causes envy or doubt is not what God sees in the heart of all men. The enemy tricks us and lies to us about others having it easy and so we will begin the big pity party and lose sight of God in the trouble.*

*Then Jesus says the profound ending – don't miss it. God alone (not with your help or your control or your assistance) has overcome the world. He's giving us the last page of the book before we ever have to read it or live out the trouble. He has overcome it. He has overcome this Lyme. He has overcome. Don't focus on the trouble, focus on God. Focus on his promises; focus on the end, the resolve. He has overcome.*

*"There is a time for everything and a season for every activity under the heavens: a time to be born and a time to die.....a time to kill and a time to heal......a time to tear down and a time to build..... A time to weep and a time to laugh....A time to mourn and a time to dance." Ecc 3:2-4*

Sara Groves has a song called "What do I know" about an 88 year old friend who is afraid of dying. The song wrestles with faith at a young age, faith at an old age and what do we really know about dying. She ends the song with this "But I know to be absent from this body is to be present with the Lord, and from what I know of him, that must be pretty good."

I'm so tired of the "mourn" part of this season of life and so look forward to the "dance". Oh, I will dance again – I will dance a jig, but first I have to prevent a stroke.

# 10

## The Tug of Despair

*For my part I call illness the touchstone of the spirit, for it is then*
*that the true virtue of a man is discovered.*
*St. Al Phonsus*

A few years ago we set off on a 23 hour road trip from Wichita, KS to Ocean Isle, North Carolina with an 18 month old and a three year old. Crazy, I know, but new parents tend to be, it's what keeps it interesting. Somewhere in South Carolina about two thirds of the way, we stopped at a rest stop for bathrooms and a picnic lunch. Middle of the afternoon, humid and not a stitch of wind in sight, it had to be nearing 95 degrees at least.

Now, there is no scratch and sniff in this story, but with just the heat alone and your memories, imagine what the rest stop bathroom smelled like and how stifling to stand inside. My husband took my son and I took my daughter. There was a huge line and the changing table was set up almost as a stage for this audience that stood in the stifling heat and stench to use the facilities. It was on this stage that upon opening my daughter's heaving landfill of a diaper.

Then we got to get in line so I could go to the bathroom, but my daughter removed of her weight, she got a renewed sense of exploration. As I am dismounting from the "hover" over the stool with one hand still on the child, I hear a huge splash and clink and a simultaneous revving of the potty engine.

All this happens so fast I cannot even tell you how fast, but in an instant I turned and grabbed the culprit of the clink – our car keys. A long skinny whistle quivers in my hand, as the giant overbearing power engine of the rest stop bathroom auto flushes and begins to pull the keys down the toilet. Still in a compromised pants down position and still holding my daughter with one hand, I am pulling with all the strength I have to keep our vacation, our entire sacrifice for the journey from being in vain. While I am fighting for my life to keep hold of those keys in the described position, the blast from this powerful flush (why is it so strong?) is causing the water to splash back all over my arm, hand, shirt, face and hair.

I don't know how long I held on and pulled against that evil flusher, but I did come out victorious. We kept the keys and continued the vacation. And the long line of people who got to see and experience the stinky poop changing diaper got to see me walk out wet from the incident. You have no idea what the look on my husband's face was like when he saw us. After I cleaned up and changed my shirt it took miles for me to be able to talk about it and years before I could have laughed about it.

One of my heart friends in MO bought me a wristlet for my keys that I have to this day. That wristlet is the best investment she could have ever made for me. But I wonder, through Lyme disease, what are you going to fasten yourself to?

In this pit, in this valley, in this disease, hold tight to hope - to Christ - to joy, to life like I held those keys. Hold tight and fight against the power flusher that is trying to destroy your ability to live. The enemy power flusher is trying to take your courage, eliminate your joy and rain on your parade of life. Hold tight to Jesus and fight to keep hold no matter how long it takes and what you get hit in the face with.

Even the new wristlet has meaning. Because there are times in this fight you feel you haven't the strength to hold on, but if you affix your faith and attach yourself to Jesus, you will remain steady. Wear Him each day, carry Him with you. If you've ever played tug of war, picture it in your mind. If you are the back person for the team, you must plant your feet, dig in and lean back expecting the tug and pull to catapult you forward. This health battle is a tug of war, and all-out war, not just for your physical body but for your soul. Will you give up in despair and begin blaming God or will you praise him and lean into Him? Dig in your feet, anchor to Him who can withstand the tugging and pulling. Brace against the Rock of Ages.

After four months of this constant tug-and pull through healing, God provided some relief. I was feeling stronger for moments, days, but the pressure in my chest and throbbing in my head was getting worse.

I travelled to Las Vegas through exhausting layovers and wheelchairs, still too weak to walk very far. An MRI revealed that my left jugular was almost completely blocked and my right was partially. These results confirmed what the doctors in

Wichita initially inferred, I had Chronic Cerebrospinal Venous Insufficiency (CCSV) I and needed to schedule intervention. Surging into my brain and unable to come out, blood was "backsliding" back down the arteries and causing immense pressure against my heart. Not only causing pain, pressure, and arrhythmias, this condition also increased brain fog, memory loss and confusion.

As I had been getting better from the Lyme perspective and my body had been getting stronger, my energy level had increased. With increased energy comes increased blood flow, except that I still had a huge blockage. It would be like a flooded river coming up to a dam, without the proper water release through the dam, the dam could burst from the pressure.

By the grace of God, they had a cancellation and I was returned by plane in a few short weeks to have the procedure done. Now, I don't know about you, but having surgery that relates to my heart and my brain was terrifying for me. Certain this intervention would be pivotal in my healing, it still felt like a terrific obstacle to pass through.

As I felt better and stronger at times, the blood flow issues, headaches, chest pressure, arrhythmia, got increasingly worse. I couldn't lay down flat at all without tremendous pain and throbbing occurring. I knew in the depths of my soul, the jugular blockage was a dam that could burst from the pressure of the blood flow against it.

Before I departed for the surgery, I wrote letters to my husband and both kids. Just in case letters – only they didn't feel just in case. When you are standing at death's door, you keep expecting it to usher you on through at any moment. Tear droplets stained all three letters, at the very idea that I wouldn't make it back from Vegas.

Leaving my family behind, a friend travelled to Nevada again with me through the airport wheelchair fiascos to face unclogging the blood from my jugulars and brain. Two days prior to surgery, the doctor ran an additional MRI to check a concern he had, a calcified blood clot in my left back sinus drainage. How long it had been there I don't know. Maybe a sports injury or car wreck, but my body had already "rerouted" blood flow around that injury. Since my left jugular was almost completely blocked, there was literally no exit for the blood to leave my left brain. None at all. No wonder I felt so terrible.

Then I began to ponder and listen to the doctor discuss the precautions they will take to break up any clots that could dislodge during or after surgery. I know how dangerous blood clots can be - deadly. How could I even process all this and continue knowing it could be the end? I couldn't handle one more thing, not one more thing. The Lord had to take this and use it for His glory, because I couldn't fathom surviving it.

At this point, anesthesia sounds like a good rest – but no. I had to be awake and cognizant during the procedure. Awake and talking to the surgeon to move my head, to answer how do you feel, etc. all to ensure the procedure was successful. Really? This almost sent me over the edge. Somehow it seemed an easy out to slowly fall asleep so I couldn't worry or have anxiety about it.

Remarkably, the morning of the procedure I had peace without loss of sensation. Only God can do that.

The parable of the wise and foolish builders applies here (Matthew 7:24-27). If your house is built on the rock, it doesn't matter what the enemy hits you with and it doesn't matter how strong the blast is. Your house will stand. Claiming God as my source of strength and guidance, my house was strong and could withstand the hits.

This is a journal entry from a 17 year old patient from the Lyme clinic I met and her courage needs no introduction:

*We are SO blessed*

*So tonight I have just been thinking about so many things. I don't know if ya'll realize it but we all have SO many blessings in our life. I think that many people don't fully realize how blessed they are because they are focusing on what is wrong in their life and what other people have that they don't have. Now I could be completely wrong, but I know that when I got sick, that's all I could focus on. Correct me if I'm wrong, but when a lot is going wrong in your life you tend to focus on the negative, yes?*

*The past couple months I have realized how AMAZING God is and how He blesses us each in our own way. I think it is amazing how he brings people in and out of your life as HE sees fit. Looking back a couple months ago, when I lost many of my friends, I NEVER thought that good could come out of that. I mean, who would?! But now, as months have gone by, He has brought SO many people into my life that have changed it dramatically for the better.*

*I know for me, when I first got sick, I felt abandoned by God or like he was punishing me for something I did. I have really spent a lot of time praying and reading my Bible and every single time, I would feel God telling me "Hold on a little bit longer. Good will come out of this I promise. I have not forgotten you or forsaken you. You are MY child, MY beloved gem, and I am always by your side". This is the first time I have ever told anyone that before. A verse that ALWAYS comes to mind when I'm feeling discouraged is Isaiah 41:10 and it says: So do not fear, for I am with you; do not be dismayed, for I am your God. I will strengthen you and help you; I will uphold you with my righteous right hand.*

*Some times in the middle of our little mess, we forget how BIG we're blessed.*

*Caity - 17*

What does it take to have that kind of strength and hope in the valley? It takes Christ. A willingness to let Christ have it. So let him have it. Give it over to him and let his strength permeate your every cell. I don't know many grownups that have that kind of wisdom, that kind of depth of knowledge from the pit, let alone someone who is only 17. But that is what the valley teaches. So much of our soul grows in the valley.

### Journal Entry:

*I am lying awake again tonight unable to sleep in the illness. The CCSVI problem with blood flow out of my brain is sending my body into sheer terror and panic. How this feels is difficult to describe. Picture a garbage disposal that can't drain and backflow coming out of the dishwasher back into the sink.....all the blood that needs to be "filtered" and processed back through the heart and filtering organs is swishing back into the good blood and getting clogged up in my brain.*

*Trying to convince your mind that your body and all it is feeling will not be your ultimate demise is truly mind over matter. If I didn't know what was happening, I would be*

83

*going to the hospital for a blood clot or heart attack or something. That is why one of the biggest challenges in this illness is the fear quotient. Add the amount of ammonia and neurotoxins floating around in my brain to the bad cloggy blood and you will understand why having any rational thought process and beating down the fear is virtually impossible. Brain fog doesn't even begin to explain how hard it is to think and get from A to B, let alone to C or D.*

*In these late night moments, the Lord will meet with me. I have felt many times in my walk with the Lord that I know His voice and can discern His leading and recognize it in my life. But actually having Him whisper to me through His own scripture is beyond amazing. Without these almost unbearable nights of pain/struggle and without the time at death's door, I would have missed this treasure in knowing Him. What I have realized though, that without consistent study and memorization of His word, He and I would have not gotten to have this kind of "talk". Oh, if I had known that all the healthy time I could have prepared even more so I could have had more to "listen" to from His word.*

*As the pain and panic rise, I pray for the Lord to bring me peace and carry me through another episode. Don't get me wrong, I'm no saint; I also beg it to be taken away, to be healed and show His glory in it. And I beg for this to be the last one, for the moments to end. But then hearing His voice say, "Have I not commanded you? Be strong and courageous, do not be terrified, do not be discouraged for the Lord your God will be with you wherever you go." Joshua 1:9*

*Hours later, I am praying that if this one does take my life, that he will provide abundantly for my husband and kids – comfort them in their loss and remain close to him and never doubt His faithfulness or plan in having to lose their mother. And He answers me again, "All the days of your life were ordained for you before even one of them came to pass." Psalm 139: 16*

*Why me, I cry out to Him, Lord, why this? Couldn't I have learned this lesson another way? He answers me "You are fearfully and wonderfully made....when I was woven together in the depths of the earth, just my eyes saw your unformed body." Psalm 139:14*

*Finally in exhaustion, I pray for it to pass and for sleep to come and he reminds me to claim his promise "My presence will go with you and I will give you rest." Exodus 33:14*

To triumph in the valley does not necessarily mean I've gotten to the mountaintop. Triumph in this valley will look different to each of us, but it remains the same inside. It becomes a state of mind. It is a soul balancing recognition that the valley and mountaintop are not the point. It is the grace in which we proceed through them that counts. Remember the verse in Joshua 1:9 – it is a command to be strong and courageous.

# 11

## Go to the Sea

*He has chosen not to heal me, but to hold me. The more intense the pain, the closer His embrace.*
*- Joni Eareckson Tada*

Near the end of the second Narnia film 'Prince Caspian', Peter, Edmund, Susan, Prince Caspian and the Narnians are backed up against a hill and pinned down by an enemy that has them outnumbered and outmaneuvered. Lucy has gone into the woods in search of Aslan the lion to help them in this plight. As they turn to consider retreat, their only exit becomes blocked. They look back to the horizon one more time to see if there is any sign of Lucy or Aslan or any help. There is none in sight.

No matter how many times I see it, I get goosebumps and, of course, tears because I always get tears. The kids turn back to the enemy and with only glances between them; unspoken looks of courage, they pull their swords and charge back at the enemy. They attack in spite of immense odds. Everyone would tell them it was futile, people would understand surrender I'm sure. But it takes bravery for them to not just stay in the battle, but to charge. To attack.

Moments after this brave attack, reinforcements come and chase the enemy back. Then God shows up in their flank to crush their leaders and send the entire army to surrender. Don't we all love a hero who choses courage against all odds?

Don't you think, based on biblical examples, that this is what God expects from us in the face of an overwhelming enemy? Muster all the courage one could gather and just say "not today" and attack it. Attack it with all you have, joy, strength, prayer - everything you've got in the arsenal. Don't hold back if you want to gain the victory.

Have you done this Lymie? Have you used all you have in the arsenal for one more frontal attack with everything you've got? Have you listened for what He is asking you to do? Is it to have a full heart of thanksgiving? Is it to praise him in joyful celebration? Is it to have courage to make a plan for tomorrow, or the courage not to? Something, no matter how insignificant not matter how small, can make a difference.

*"Have faith in God," Jesus answered. "Truly I tell you, if anyone says to this mountain, 'Go, throw yourself into the sea,' and does not doubt in their heart but believes that what they say will happen, it will be done for them. Therefore I tell you, whatever you ask for in prayer, believe that you have received it, and it will be yours." (Mark 11:22-25)*

There is power in believing.

*"Because you have so little faith, truly I tell you, if you have faith as small as a mustard see, you can say to this mountain, "move from here to there" and it will move. Nothing will be impossible for you. Truly I tell you, if you have faith and do not doubt, not only can you do what was done to the fig tree, but also you can say to this mountain, go throw yourself into the sea and it will be done." (Matthew 17:20-21)*

If Jesus said it then we can believe it.

Oh, you don't know how many times, I cast this health crisis in the sea. "To the sea, to the sea" I would scream and cry out in the shower, in the tub, in the car. TO THE SEA! I cast it out still. I cast out the remnants, the leftover damage. Then I began to start thanking him. I couldn't feel it gone yet, I couldn't feel anything change. But since one day is a thousand to the Lord and a thousand days are as one day. I thanked him for doing it. I thanked Him that he heard me and that he gave me a faith so strong to believe.

In Joshua chapter 3, the Israelites are preparing to cross the Jordan River and began laying claim to the Promised Land but the river is in flood stage. Out of obedience, Joshua commands the priests carrying the ark to step in the flood stage river to cross because the Lord has promised he would stop the water. Not before they cross, not when they get close. But when they take that first step into the raging river.

After an action of obedience, he stops the flow of river until all the people cross. In similar fashion, he can stop Lyme too.

*"But I trust in you, Lord, I say, you are my God. My times are in your hands; deliver me from the hands of my enemies, from those who pursue me." (Psalm 31:14-15)*

Mark Batterson has a mantra he repeats often in his book "The Circle Maker" –"work like it depends on you and pray like it depends on God." We can get caught up in the waiting upon the Lord and miss the opportunity for action. In our action sometimes the pathway opens up. Our first steps take us to a whole other realm of healing and spiritual understanding. Taking the first steps give us the courage to take another.

In Batterson's book 'In a Pit with a Lion on a Snowy Day', he says one of my favorite phrases of all time. Read it twice to let it sink in. "God wants you to get where God wants you to go more than you want to get where God wants you to go."

Let that one marinate a bit longer. As much as we want to continue on with life and be a better person at the end of this illness, God wants that for us even more. In fact, He doesn't want us to wait until the end to improve. He seeks that for us even now in the valley and in the suffering.

In "In a Pit with a Lion on a Snowy Day" Batterson (I could quote him all day, but will try to keep it down to a few times a chapter) says "God is in the resume building business. He is always using past experiences to prepare us for future opportunities but those God given opportunities often come disguised as man-eating lions."

Take heart, hear and remember: God loves to rescue out of the lion's den. He loves to stop the flow of the river after we step. If He played football, God would be in the Hail Mary pass into the end zone. If God was in basketball it would be for the full court shot at the buzzer. It gives Him glory. It removes our ability to claim we did anything, takes our pride out of the equation. It shows off His miracles, His power and gives Him the ultimate credit.

*"Praise be to the Lord, who has given rest to his people just as he promised. Not one word has failed of all the good promises he gave through his servant Moses." (1 Kings 8:56)*

*"Through these he has given us his very great and precious promises, so that through them you may participate in the divine*

*nature, having escaped the corruption in the world caused by evil desires." (2 Peter 1:4)*

Go ahead and try one of these promises on for size. Put your name and your singular pronouns in the blanks below and let it soak into your heart over and over again.

Jeremiah 31:2-4 This is what the Lord says, "_____ who survive the sword (this illness) will find favor in the wilderness; I will come to give rest to _____. The Lord appeared to _____ in the past saying I have loved you with an everlasting love; I have drawn you with unfailing kindness, I will build you up again and your _____will be rebuilt. Again you will take out your timbrels and go out to dance with the joyful."

### *Journal Entry:*

*I am trying to get over a hump that remains a mountain. I've cast this burden to the sea. I believe, I've been thankful, I've been faithful, I trust and here the hump remains.*

*An obstacle, casting a dark shadow of discouragement upon my soul today. I scream at the vast impending hump "not today – I demand the sunlight not your shadow. I will climb you, walk around you or tear you down but not today will I be in your shadow." But still it looms before me.*

*My devotional entitled "the great escape" shared this verse this day that I so desperately needed. "Oh that I had the wings of a dove, I would fly away and be at rest." Psalm 55:6*

*Fly over the dadgum hump of a mountain – only on the spirit's wings and only He could design such a beautiful thing as flight over it, instead of trudging through it or around it or trying to move it. To fly above it and see it as a small insignificant thing to overcome as He sees it.*

91

*I trust you Lord to pick me up and fly me over in your time. Until then, I will rest in the shadow of your wing and not the shadow of your hump until this calamity has passed me by.*

After the CCSVI surgery, the next morning I woke up and felt FANTASTIC! More fantastic than I had felt in years. I told my friend "let's get dressed and eat and go to Red Rock Canyon". I was ready to sightsee. In the tug and pull of Lyme, I had already learned that when you have a window of strength, you had to seize it and make the most of it. Most people said, oh take it easy and don't over do it. But Lymie, remember, the good days are surrounded by bad days. Make the most of the good days. Go and do and live and then patiently wait for another good day to come. They will come.

One of the doctors told me "the good days will get longer and come more often. It happens slowly, but it does happen."

So off we went to Red Rock Canyon. I had a wonderful morning driving and taking pictures at the marvel of that place. Just as we were finishing up our morning by going into the visitor center to get souvenirs for my kids, a wall hit me with a vengeance. I almost passed out from the sheer darkness and heaviness of it. Bam! Just like that I was down again.

# 12

**This is Your Life**

*I will stand and wholly say, this is my life.*
*Jeremy Camp (song)*

This journey through life/Lyme can be compared to going down a giant waterslide. The drops, curves and tunnels are brushes with death - the worst of times - but the anticipation for the end and knowing that, no matter what happens, I'm on the waterslide. I'm not leaving the slide until the end has been designated. It's not a get-off-the-ride-early kind of ride. I might get higher on some curves and get more scared of the heights or get more wet than someone else, but we will all reach the end eventually. The end, the wonderful climax of being dumped and immersed in the pool at the end.

When we are on the waterslide with God, He serves as the living water that keeps it going, prevents us from getting stuck and immerses us once the journey is complete. The slide wouldn't work without water – we flow much smoother through the trials and tribulations of this world with God carrying us along the journey.

When we were kids and went to a waterpark once, I remember these particular older kids would try to get stuck in one of the curves until they had a dangerous pileup to go down together. They would send the biggest kid down and he would jam his feet against the sides pushing against the water pressure to hold there until all his friends had slammed into him, creating a catastrophic pileup.

Isn't that what we do in a trial, when we dig in to fear, frustration and discouragement? Instead of trusting and releasing to the Lord through it and "rolling with it", we dig in our heels, rest in our fear/pain and fight the current rushing down on us. We know the ride is not over but maybe somehow, by holding position in the middle of the ride, we can change the outcome, change what will happen next. We fight against the Lord when we say, why me, why this?

Instead of thanking Him for it and knowing that He who allowed this or sifted me through this, is also the maker of the heavens and the earth. He cradles and carries me down in the water to be immersed in His pool. Whether the immersion pool at the end of your waterslide is the grace of the mountaintop of healing, or is heaven itself – both are completely and utterly immersed in the Lord's presence.

I've always wondered what the Olympic luge riders felt on their "slide". I would assume it's mainly exhilaration or they wouldn't choose to do such a dangerous sport. Put me on one of those things and no matter how much I think I'm an adventure junkie, it would be sheer terror and agony, resulting in many broken pieces. So the experience of riding down many times makes the luge rider trust the equipment, trust their body's reactions, trust their coach and trust the fundamental laws of physics.

Without experience and knowledge, fear will triumph. Knowing God and trusting in His promises is the foundation of that knowledge. Then with each trial and ride down a treacherous slide, we get more and more certain of Him and the results. We can trust they will be good, because He says they will.

I know something else that luge riders do. They remember. They remember the track; they recall what their coach told them. They think of the mistakes they made and correct them to prevent an accident. They also learn the path of least resistance.

We must remember. We must evoke and call to memory His promises, His blessings, His faithfulness. Remembering builds the gumption behind a courageous charge uphill. Remembering structures the attitudes of our heart from which all actions are revealed. Lack of resistance is complete and gives way to utter obedience.

*"But we have this treasure in jars of clay to show that this all-surpassing power is from God and not from us. We are hard pressed on every side, but not crushed; perplexed, but not in despair, persecuted, but not abandoned, struck down, but not destroyed. We always carry around in our body the death of Jesus, so that the life of Jesus may also be revealed in our body. For we who are alive are always being given over to death for Jesus' sake, so that his life may also be revealed in our mortal body. So then, death is at work in us, but life is at work in you."* *(2 Corinthians 4:7)*

Like in Narnia, I picture the kind of courage I want my kids to exude in the face of fear and overwhelming odds against them. I want them to well up all they have and charge at it with all they've got. Better to try their best and lose than to live in fear. People around you are watching to see if you have what it takes in there – not simply fight back – but to charge. Is your belief in God that kind of belief?

In John Ortberg's book "If You are Going to Walk on Water, You've Got to Get Out of the Boat" he records some typical statistics of people and how they respond to trauma in their lives. The people who are marked by "resiliency", a condition in which they enlarge their capacity to handle problems and not only survive but grow.

- Resilient people continually seek to reassert some command and control over their destiny rather than seeing themselves as passive victims.
- Resilient people have a larger than usual capacity for what might be called moral courage – for refusing to betray their values
- Resilient people find purpose and meaning in their suffering

When you make your move, when you well up your courage, keep your focus on Jesus. We can courageously charge and end up crashing because we attempt by our own merits, by our own plan and with our own strength. John Ortberg points out that in the face of trauma, like Peter did when he stepped out into the raging sea and walked toward the Lord. He was doing great until "he saw the wind".

Don't look at the wind in your life after you take that step in courage. Don't listen to others telling you to take it easy, don't do too much, and don't go too fast. People telling you "I don't blame you for lying in bed". Don't give audience to naysayers about your treatment or special diet or medical expenses. After all, Solomon proved that chasing after the wind was the epitome of empty frustration.

If you have prayed over this, the Lord is guiding you. Trust His instruction when you have his permission to step out of the boat and face the raging disease of Lyme with courage. Then take a step, without looking back, without looking down. Stay focused on God. He is one that commands the laws of physics, He is the one who commands the storm to be quiet and it stills.

Listen to that still small voice and charge.

*"Sin is always a substitute for legitimate suffering. It is an attempt to obtain pleasure that does not rightly belong to me or to evade the pain that does." Carl Jung*

Oh, read that one again. Don't sin and wallow in this valley. Give up on the pity party, give up on the 'cannot' and focus on the 'can'. There might not be much that you can do, but thank Him for it and take one more step. Tell Him you are ready to fight and ask permission to walk on the water. Don't seek to satiate the flesh by dwelling on it and by avoiding the hard stuff. Take it head on.

Take that step, listen to the Lord beckon and feel it when he ignites the fire of courage in your belly.

If God sifts everything for me, and allowed this Lyme, then I cannot be disappointed with my life. Where I am and what I am fighting, He has chosen for me. Being ashamed of my life means being ashamed of Christ himself. This is my life. This is your life. Are you going to take it in the chin and go down, or give it all you've got?

This is my life, this is your life. This Lyme, this raging river of Lyme that cuts and drowns and swallows up whole. No wishing, no wondering, no looking back and no amount of pity will change it. Address the physicality of it but do not yield to its attempts to diminish you. This is your life.

### *Journal Entry:*

*I am 6 months from ground zero of diagnosis and treatment and 10 months into being chronically ill. I have undergone treatment and am feeling "better" but still fighting for my life. The kids started VBS this week at church which is great for them to get out away from me and jump for joy and be unhindered.*

*It is not such a good week for me. I am grappling and struggling, crying and just barely holding on again.*

*As I sit in the back of the gym I watch the end of the dance and song time, ready for pickup, blending in with the wall and tears were pouring out of my eyes. Not sobbing, but a silent river of tears flowing out at the amount of energy and joy in the room. How much I want to dance and feel that river of joy!*

*I look around the room and see the happy moms and happy helpers form into cliques and talk about mundane things, plan lunch dates and existing in a layer of social existence right now that I find appalling and foreign. I am unable to speak that language. I am offended with myself that I cannot relate for even a split second.*

*Do they know that their health that allows them to be helpers and mommies today is a gift I would pay in dividends for even one day again? It has been so long to have a normal thought or normal moment that I want to scream at them for being selfish, for being so normal, for being so unaware of my pain.*

*I hear it as I write it, my complaining, my pity party. Why shouldn't they enjoy their normal? Why shouldn't they live life to the full? Why shouldn't they continue in life's routine unobstructed? They don't need to throw a party with my pity any more that they need to throw a party for my new normal accomplishments. How many of these women will understand the accomplishment of doing laundry or making the beds again? How many horns will toot out exuberance that I drove my own kids again today to church? How many congratulations will I get for making our supper or going to the grocery store by myself?*

I know three other people that have had actual brain surgery. As much as I can acknowledge that no one had to actually enter my skull, my surgery was no less serious or important. Without it, my brain was clogged, unable to work and my heart would have soon failed from the pressure. But somehow, to me, my intervention was downplayed and misunderstood. Most people just got caught up in what on earth would she go to Las Vegas when we have qualified doctors here. Others who felt that Lyme wasn't that serious probably thought we were just overreacting or making it up.

I had to reconcile all of this "not feeling important" through the whole process of healing. I felt like I had an illegal illness that we couldn't talk about or acknowledge out loud. My husband and I both felt we were constantly defending our treatment plan and the expenses of it to family and friends. We have such a human need to be understood and sympathized with through trial.

Since we know no one who have travelled this road, we had no one to understand it with us. It takes brave acceptance. Courageously "moving on" to get past the culture of "no one gets it". Being part of a Lyme community was our saving grace.

One of the patients I met at Hansa called me the night before my Las Vegas procedure and walked me through it. God provided someone who knew exactly what I was facing and understood and sympathized and gave me hope. God is good all the time.

# 13

## Unglamorous Obstacles

*A restless mind can never give answers. Trust the Lord.*
*(Missionary on The Open Road)*

As a self-proclaimed recovering control freak, you might understand why I don't like riding horses. An animal bigger than me that I cannot fully control puts me at a huge disadvantage. But my sense of adventure keeps me doing and experiencing things I'd sometimes rather not. I'll try anything once, especially if competing against others for adventure points.

So I find myself on a horse for the first time at 21 years old in Wales with a group of friends on a cliff/beach trail ride. Some of you equine experts will scoff and say trail riding isn't really riding because those horses know the trail. It requires no real skill to guide them and ride. Well, I beg to differ. I believe, for the novice, it takes more proficiency to make these trail horses do anything thereby convincing them they are not in charge.

I find myself on a horse more stubborn than myself called Philly. Philly didn't mind me at first and on the uphill to the cliff top, she slowed a bit letting many of the other horses pass along. I wasn't bothered by her lack of enthusiasm, as long as we didn't fall so far behind that I lost sight of the others. Once at the top of the cliff however, Philly took a turn for the worse. On the downhill steep rocky path, she developed a front limp. Not a slight limp, but at the severe downhill angle we were traversing, I almost pitched over her head and neck more than a few times.

With my lack of experience on horses, I was certain that she had picked up a briar, a thorn, lost a horseshoe or something to exhibit this extreme behavior. Her condition persisted until we finally leveled out at the cliff bottom and came to the open meadow – which must have been secret code for RUN.

Philly took off like lightning, passing many of the horses we had fallen behind like Secretariat winning the Triple Crown. Not a limp in sight. After our wild dash, we began the trail ride through the forest back to the stables.

As you may have guessed, the limp came back even more severe on the last part of the trail. I thought I was going to fall off or we weren't going to make it. Then before me I see all the other horses slowly stepping over a large log covering the trail. How on earth will this limp and stubborn fickle horse ever make it over that big ole log?

Well, to my complete amazement the limp and fickle horse approached the log and jumped it. Yes, she jumped it. The only horse in the pack. Then she promptly limped the rest of the way back to the stable. Am I a reflection of this headstrong trailnag? Heedless of style or proper motivation?

How do I handle the unglamorous obstacles in my life? Do I charge up the mountain because it feels nostalgic and victorious, but stumble down the rocky outcropping on the other side? Do I sprint across the meadow and limp down the trail? When the

102

Lord gives me a calm in the storm, is that the only time I sprint for glee unabandoned?

If you haven't figured it out by now, Lyme is unglamorous and unpopular and quasi-understood disease. Not many do 5K walks and runs to raise money for Lyme research. There aren't any special colored ribbons you can wear or bracelets you can buy. (Well there haven't been until recently and it is still obscure) Few even know anyone whose become sick from Lyme. Most doctors just glaze over and try to give you antidepressants, circumventing true treatment. I don't mean this disparagingly for people who suffer other ailments and "popular" chronic illness. But hear me clearly, Lyme is not famous. People don't "get it."

Are you going to be fickle in this illness only gravitating toward the glamorous parts of the trail? Or are you going to hit your stride the entire journey and finish strong? These questions aren't meant rhetorically. Your response is critical to manage the duration.

The ammonia from the Lyme was deeply embedded in my pituitary gland affecting swelling against my optic nerve, so I couldn't drive or go most places. My eyes just did not function right at all. Reading and the computer were very difficult. I could watch movies or TV for a little while, but anything with text or words made my head just hurt terribly. I handled the not reading part with great stride. I am an avid reader – voracious reader, but due to the exhaustion, I just accepted this setback as part of the journey. But take away my ability to drive and you robbed me of freedom......

I did not handle this obstacle in my life with any grace. I couldn't drive myself or the kids anywhere for almost 18 months and it nagged and bugged me like crazy. I snapped at my husband and was terribly ungrateful and rude at times to some of the generous loved ones and friends who carted me everywhere. I felt so helpless, so trapped, so sheltered, so weak and dependent.

Needing help with the laundry, the dishes, the cooking, etc chipped away at my sense of independence. Needing to be wheel-chaired through an airport a humbling experience but necessary because I couldn't walk, but the loss of driving devastated my insides and caused me such turmoil. One day in particular, my husband was going to pick up my son from school – a 20 minute drive across town. He hit something metal and had a tire blow out halfway there. I had to scramble one of my "drivers" to hurry over and pick up my son. I frantically paced the front door praying and festering with worry over my son thinking we forgot him and how helpless I was to not be the rescuer. It was definitely not glamorous. Like Philly, I limped and dragged my feet through this one not accepting it and letting it tear me up.

Professionals may have told you that after a few rounds of antibiotics you would be just fine. Back to normal. Back in the saddle. The trail ride is longer than that and the terrain is rough-

and-tumble. Don't we all know that now? Lyme recovery is not a sprint, it is a marathon, or an Iron Man competition.

Say you get hit by a truck. You can have surgeries and physical therapies and eventually walk again and resume all the activities you once experienced. You can recover from the accident, but people who knew you before the accident will notice a slight limp. Or the guys you play basketball with on Saturdays will notice the knee brace and that you are a bit slower getting down the court. Your spouse will notice you are more reluctant to mow the lawn and get tired faster. There are scars left behind and the range of motion has been reduced.

How about a car that has an accident? The title becomes a salvage title, always to be sold for less, never to be worth the same, never to be made whole again no matter how well she runs or looks. That label is forever emblazoned on that title as a scarlet letter of shame for what it has physically experienced. So it is for the Lyme body – stamped with the disease, ever to be affected by it. Never the same. Ever stamped with the disease's scarlet letter "L" on the forehead – designating the damage left from Lyme.

Yes, you recover, you resume but are you back to normal? Navigating the new normal in Lyme carries in baggage that has to be unpacked. Unpacked by a counselor, a pastor, a friend, a spouse (who might also need to have baggage unpacked with help).

What is left? What has changed? What can and can't you do now? Some changes are subtle and some are vast. They are different for us all.

### *Journal Entry:*

*In the New Normal my physical body still feels like aliens have taken it over and only half of them got the eviction notice. The other half has every intention of being those tenants that leave a path of trash in their wake and upon their exit, give Jeff Foxworthy enough jokes about rednecks for a year – leaving cars on blocks, TVs on the porch and laundry in the front lawn.*

*For women, you will understand it as a close analogy to being pregnant. Your body is not your own anymore, what you used to know about it is completely different. I am starting all over again to feel and learn its idiosyncrasies.*

*Sitting in Bible study this morning there are half a dozen things that I feel going on in my body that are not normal and I do not recall feeling or experiencing before this disease. I began to process through them and try to do the mental gymnastics it takes to suppress my panicked mind from taking any of these warning bells too seriously:*

- *Thick and swollen tongue*
- *Heart and chest feeling tight*
- *Throat feels constricted*
- *Dull ache in right ear*
- *Light headed and slightly dizzy*
- *Unable to properly focus eyes*

*Now am I just uber aware of my physical body and slightly paranoid or are things still misfiring and not normalized because half of the aliens are still illegally squatting in this physical shell?*

*Another Lyme patient told me recently she understands what it feels like to be her 92 year old mother (although she would never tell her that) because of being trapped against*

106

*your will inside a failing physical body, like being in a straightjacket, but you still have full mental faculties.*

*Even the brain fog days feel like a straightjacket because it's like there is the quiet, smart person hidden deep inside there, but they have been put in the very back of the house down a long hallway and have food in their mouth so you can hardly hear them let alone understand them. You know that smart person is there and would know just where you put your keys or the kid's homework and how to balance the bank account, but you just cannot make out the instructions through the quiet muffled voice.*

*Good news! "I have been crucified with Christ and I no longer live, but Christ lives in me. The life I now live in the body, I live by faith in the Son of God, who loved me and gave himself for me." (Galatians 2:20)*

Good news! What hasn't changed? Christ lived in my body pre-Lyme and Christ resides in me still post-Lyme. This life I now live in the body can still be lived by faith in the Son of God. What else hasn't changed? His promises, His hope, His goodness.

*"Forget the former things; do not dwell on the past. See, I am doing a new thing? Now it springs up; do you not perceive it? I am making a way in the wilderness and streams in the wasteland." Isaiah 43:18-19*

Unglamorous obstacles cannot hinder me from the life God wants to give me. I choose to live by faith and leap when necessary.

# 14

## Last Call – The Pity Party is Over

*A single sunbeam is enough to drive away many shadows.*
*- St. Francis of Assisi*

While undergoing Lyme therapy I ran into a patient from Maryland for the second time. This is one of the many blessings God gave me on my Lyme journey - other Lymies with which to share the success and pain. I recognize her right away sitting in one of the therapy rooms.

Claudette* began sharing her struggle in flying here alone through a layover, all the while feeling so terrible and weak. Awesome moment. I take the opportunity to to "ohh and ahh" her ability to achieve such an amazing feat for a Lymie. This is quite an accomplishment and feels like to me she just won the Iditarod Dog Sled race. The infamous Iditarod Dog Sled race that was named after a dog named Balto and was deemed 'indefatigable' and 'indomitable'. We understand this to be more of a term of 'never give up' attitude that leads to the impossible.

While she was sitting exhausted and discouraged in her layover, she began watching all the people scurrying around the busy airport. She saw herself, the former professional traveler, the high powered business suit heading off to another city, another agenda, another meeting, another mountain to climb. Previously, self-absorbed, busy, on the phone, hurrying along and here she was sitting barely able to hold her head up being pushed in a wheelchair to her gate. She began to weep and weep, mourning the loss of that person. That person she felt she would never be again.

She cried out to God "why this and why me?" We began to cry together because this is one of those moments my tear ducts are not going to pass up joining in the crying party. I knew exactly how that moment felt, anyone in chronic illness does. That person she was, that person I was. That person you have been. They are gone, never to return. Like a soldier that goes off to war and survives battle but comes home transformed physically and emotionally. Like the mother that loses her stillborn baby, a husband widowed – we will never be the same again.

God uses adversity and weakness to build us up or shape us into better people. Or, as in my case, to tear down bad things within us that we didn't even realize were festering. In the movie "French Kiss" with Meg Ryan, her character is making fun of Kevin Kline's character, Luke, who is scowling and pouting. "Fester, fester, fester, rot, rot, rot" she says to him mimicking his attitude and body language. He was going to become a cranky old man unless he shifted his attitude.

Things festering unbeknownst to me that need to be removed. I could not grow and accomplish what God had planned for me where I was. In order to handle the Promised Land He has prepared in advance for me, I had to be toughened up. Being put through some battles along the way, I learned to trust Him fully and demonstrate that I could be trustworthy.

My son's teacher once gave me a photocopy of a devotional that told about how soldiers are prepared for battle. How do they become better? More skilled? By drills and practice or actual battle field experience? Good generals and commanders are shaped in the heat of battle, in the heat of many battles.

So the Lord drills us, drills our lives with circumstances intended to build experiences.

In my tattered and worn copy of 31 Days of Praise, day 31 reads, "You who began a good work in me will carry it to completion until the day of Christ Jesus. You are utterly faithful and will finish what you have set out to do. So I need not stagger at your promises or waver in unbelief" (Philippians 1:6)

*"Blessed is the Lord.....according to all that he promised; not one word has failed for all his good promises." (I Kings 8:56)*

The enemy has tried to defeat me all the time with "I deserved this sickness" because of my lack of faith. Or was it my lack of fruit or my selfishness? Maybe a consequence of my rebellious past was catching up with me. He used people around me to subtly suggest this was a consequence of my sin, my past, my disobedience. As ultimate blame, the enemy loves to say – it's because of a lack of faith on my part or a lack of faithfulness from God himself.

Yet I am reminded that because of my faith, not a lack thereof, God began a good work in me despite my failings not because of them. And He who began this good work, plans on

111

finishing it up because he planned it in advance just for me (Eph 2:10) The completion of good work is part of God's character.

With or without my cooperation He intends to fulfill that promise. As I tell my kids in a clash of wills, they can stop and think about this and do it the hard way or the easy way, but it is going to happen regardless of what they choose.

Who would choose the hard way? I would. I have. I do still. But learn from me and don't repeat it for yourself. Don't fight God's promises or His plan. Just get on board. Chose the easy way early on, accept it and move on. This sets the new normal into place. Don't look back. The going might still be difficult, but who would chose to move forward without Him, outside his will? I cannot imagine what the hard way would look like in this valley, but I would be incapable alone.

The surrender of my will, allows me to choose the easy way with the Lord. Easy, not because it won't be hard and be without struggle, but easier because I won't be fighting my will through the journey. Without true surrender, I make the easy way difficult because I am at odds with God. If I'm fickle and only surrender on the not-so-bad days, the journey can be bumpy and inconsistent. A journey that lacks continuity of will cannot be a smooth one.

In a song by Sara Groves called "painting pictures of Egypt" the chorus:

I've been painting pictures of Egypt
Leaving out what it lacked
The future seems so hard
And I want to go back

112

But the places that used to fit me
Cannot hold the things I've learned
And those roads closed off to me
While my back was turned

My favorite verse three says "The past is so tangible, I know it by heart, familiar things are never easy to discard...Caught between the promise and the things I know."

We all paint pictures of our Egypt – our past. The things we know, the places we've been, the things we remember. Lyme suffers feel like we are caught between this physical chronic illness and the promises of God. How can those reconcile? Painting pictures of the past births the pity party. It hinders us from acceptance. Is there going to be sadness? Are there going to be tears? Yes, most certainly. If tears were not allowed I would have been disqualified from this journey a long time ago. Sadness and mourning are a part of learning acceptance. They are necessary components of surrendering your will.

The flow of tears that plants and waters acceptance seeds to sprout our new belief system.

### Journal Entry:

*I am having a huge pity party today. Huge. I can't get anything accomplished. I felt great last week and thought I was cruising, onward and upward. And here I am peeling myself out of bed, too dizzy to get around and feeling just plain awful.*

*Each of these renewed crashes have me reeling in the pain and fear of going backward. I am holding on and grasping for the forward momentum and feeling like it's one step forward and two steps back.*

113

*I am prostrate crying out to God. I just want to be a mom again. I just want to be able to function to handle life again. And in one final blow I blurt out 'I wanna be that mom again, the mom I was. When am I going to be her again Lord?'*

*Audibly deep in my gut I hear "but that person was selfish and that person was ungrateful."*

*The truth hits hard. That person was terribly ungrateful and horribly selfish. Oh my, how the truth hurts and can put a serious end to a wildly successful pity party. The balloons pop, the music grinds to a halt and I realize without a shadow of doubt that I don't want to be that person again. I don't want to be that person I was before. I have no desire to be that selfish, or controlling, or ungrateful.*

*That person is gone forever, forever changed for the better through this valley.*

After the surgery in Las Vegas and the subsequent crash that followed, my body began a steady climb out of the pit. Not fast, not exceptional, but it was notably onward and upward. Incredibly frustrating at times,. I couldn't shower without getting dizzy. I needed help doing laundry and loading the dishwasher because bending over gave me a ridiculous head rush.

My body had to get used to blood flow again. The body, being the amazing creation that it is, had compensated and then the flood gate was literally released. Compare this to carrying around a 50 lb bag of flour on your left side and learning to walk, run and dance normal. Then after years of carrying the 50 lbs, it was suddenly gone. It would feel unbalanced.

Just like getting off an ocean cruise, after the CCSVI surgery, I had to find my "sea legs" again. My body had to learn

114

to walk, bend, stand, sit and balance all over again with my new blood flow. I was also learning to walk, talk and live again spiritually with my new faith.

You must be born again – no kidding.

# 15

## The New Normal

*Contentment ... has an internal quietness of heart that gladly submits to God in all circumstances.*
*Joni Eareckson Tada*

My family comes from a long line of musicians (it skipped me) on both sides and on my mom's side for generations we sing grace at family dinners. We continue the tradition in our household and often while I was sick, my daughter would chose to sing one of her favorites. I would choke up and not even be able to utter the words through my sobs. Mommy's crying again and off one of them trots to get me some Kleenex.

*"Oh the Lord is good to me and so I thank the Lord for giving me the things I need, the sun and the rain and the apple seed, Oh the Lord is good to me."*

The Lord is good to me. The Lord is good to you. Have I thanked him today for giving me the things I need? Have you? Caught every time, I'm red handed in thanklessness. He has given me the things I need. He gives the sun, the rain and the seed. He gives life and he causes ALL things to grow. All things. Everything has life because He gives.

But He alone gives the seed, the water and the sun. We must wait for it to grow and bear fruit. The seed in our lives, by watering it with the wellspring of life from Jesus will grow fruit. He knows what I need; he is good to provide just what I need. I must thank him. Therefore, gratitude becomes my automatic default.

Mark Batterson in "Drawing the Circle" says "When was the last time you thanked God for keeping the earth in its perfect orbit and spinning on its perfect axis to give us a day and a season and a year?" When was the last time you were worried God couldn't handle that and things might not just work out with the whole sunrise thing tomorrow morning? If he can handle such big things without our need to fret or fester or worry, he can handle all the little things, big things and things in between.

As I write this section during a week that God chose to put on the calendar months ago, I realize what He has done in the timing. It is holy week. Yesterday I was overcome with Maundy Thursday. The day he washed the disciple's feet. The day he broke bread and drank the cup. The day he looked Judas in the eye mere hours before the betrayal. The day he knew would be the last of the "old normal" for him and these guys. The day he entered the deepest part of the valley. The day he had been preparing for had come. NO laughter after today, no healing, no feeding, no teaching, only suffering remained for tomorrow.

Jesus himself described what he felt in the Garden as "My soul is overwhelmed with sorrow to the point of death." (Mark 14:34)

From here on friends would abandon him, crowds would crucify him, government would execute him, and even believers would disown him. He would be alone in agonizing prayer to face Friday. We ironically refer to this as Good Friday, because we know the outcome on Sunday. But to everyone involved, Friday was dark, sad, painful and full of anguish and suffering - a dark day.

A day passes and I pick up writing again on dark Friday and contemplate Christ. Where was He this time of day? Was he before Caiaphas or Pilate? How much beating had He taken already? How much betrayal and hurt did His human heart feel? How much anticipation for the pain of the cross, the battle of conquering death itself lay before Him? Each step between here and there travelled down deeper in the pit. He would get not a moment of respite today. Not a moment. He would hear his people, the people he had healed and loved and taught and came to save chant "crucify him, crucify him."

He knew the end, he knew the resurrection was coming also, but still He prayed three times in the Garden "My Father if it is possible, may this cup be taken from me. Yet not as I will but as you will." Matthew 26:39

It's okay to keep asking, to keep begging for the end to come for Lyme. I know that in your new normal it is still hard, hard to do so many things. Keep asking. Keep meeting the Lord in your trial. The days are long but the years are short. Slowly the days will come with relief, but they will come. It took me nine months to be able to read again and 15 months to be able to drive again most days. Recovery takes time.

*"I waited patiently for the Lord; he turned to me and heard my cry. He lifted me out of the slimy pit out of the mud and mire; he set my feet on a rock and gave me a firm place to stand. He put a new song in my mouth a hymn of praise to our God. Many*

119

*will see and fear the Lord and put their trust in Him. Blessed is the one who trust in the Lord.....I desire to do your will, my God, your law is within my heart." (Psalm 40:1-4, 8)*

It snowed a few weeks ago over 21 inches in less than a week. A record setting experience for southern Kansas. Here I am, nearly 18 months from ground zero of the illness and what thought pops in my mind? "What happens if it snows so much we can't get out in case I need to go to the emergency room?" There I am back to the emotion and fear of Near Death. The mindset trapped in chronically ill, not to healing and forward.

Adjusting and wishing my immediate response had been 'can't wait to take the kids outside sledding in this'. My knee jerk reaction came from my old normal – not my recovering mind. The simple act of rerouting my thoughts again needs immense concentration and recognition. I spent so many months not doing, not able to do, not sure what I could do, that to think I could almost felt criminal.

I would get so dizzy from the blood flow problems in my head while doing laundry, or the dishes, or climbing stairs, showering or taking a bath. I wouldn't do them alone or with the kids alone. I still catch myself thinking I'll wait and shower when my husband gets home. Why? Because I did it that way for so long. The mind gets in habits. The rut represents a safe place where the results are in your favor.

Do I have my cellphone? Do the kids know how to dial for emergencies? Have the neighbors gotten home from work if something happens?

The questions and the habits of living in chronic illness have to be broken one-by-one and habit-by-habit. Check your habits, which ones are you still living or thinking? What negative mindsets have taken root that the enemy is using to keep you feeling guilty or in fear? The habit that outlives its reason becomes a vice – a dangerous vice.

In the third Narnia movie, Eustace describes what it was like to have Aslan the lion (Jesus) to turn him back into a boy from a dragon. He says it hurt, but in a good way, like when you pull out a thorn. I have resisted this journey at times. We all do. We all will. Because when I am weak, I'm convincingly weak. But with Christ....I am strong. I resonate with Eustace when he says in the same scene "It wasn't bad really, I was a better dragon than I was a boy."

Am I a better sick person than I was when I was well?

### Journal Entry:

*The kids are having one of those mornings getting ready for school and I have one of those mornings getting them ready for school. Then they leave and I'm hit with this immense guilt for them leaving for school in such a state – will they question my love for them if I die today? What if that is the last time I see them? Am I being ungrateful for them and unflexible in them being kids?*

*I begged God to let me be their mom and raise them, and here I am barking orders and shooing them out the door in a rush. Shouldn't I wake up every day grateful and cheery and handle things better? How can I beg God to be here and not get things right or better? Has this experience not changed me at all?*

*Or then I think, didn't the kids get the memo about the near death experience? Shouldn't they be cutting me some slack and be more agreeable, not bickering, and being more obedient? Oyyy, the thoughts go on and on.*

*The "I have to be perfect and leave every single situation and relationship perfectly in case I'm about to die" is a HUGE vice of pressure to be in. The enemy uses every circumstance to try to trip us up in our emotive state. He loves to tear it into disarray and distrust in our maker who put us here.*

*I know that "feeling whole in case I die today" is horrible pressure to be under. I am not going to be perfect all the time whether dying or alive. Yes, we're all told not to let the sun go down on our anger and yes, this near death has impacted me greatly for the better. But unfortunately as I heal, I am still 100% carnal and sinful, I didn't get a transplant of heavenly material that has made me less so. I am no less sinful. I am just more aware of my sinful state and how I want to live differently – my will has changed, my character has grown in the refinement. But my sinful nature remains the same.*

*In fact it is the only thing from pre-Lyme that is unchanged. God help me out from under the emotional strangle-hold to be perfect to everyone all the time. My kids will disobey, my husband might forget our anniversary, and it's not about the Near Death.*

Life after Near Death – insert your disaster here – is a tricky balance beam of emotions. The enemy wages war within while we try to regain our footing in the new normal. Keep the enemy in check; do not let him get a stronghold here in fear and perfectionism. It's a landmine of intense emotions, a roller coaster and horror house willing us to engage in gratefulness, delight one moment and guilt and sheer terror the next.

Navigating the new normal is impossible in the flesh. The emotional and spiritual battle are just as thick on this Lyme thing as the physical. Sometimes I thought the emotional even harder. More mind-over-body type of thinking lays the groundwork and provides the map for how to navigate out of this thing and find a new normal, one that works for you.

The new normal is not easy and there will be times of dismal failure as you try to find your "sea legs". Follow me through the tools that helped me survive and find mine.

# 16

## Quit Looking at the Deep End

*He has always appeared for my help, I delight in speaking well of His name.*
*- George Mueller*

Last summer, my five year old daughter struggled with putting her face in the water during swimming lessons. The teacher would try her best using every technique in her arsenal, but to no avail. After a few days, we began to practice the face-in-the-water technique in the bathtub. Even blowing nose bubbles with the face plant in the tub became quite successful.

Then in swimming lessons, she would get fearful and not even try it at all. So, the next bathtub training session, I began to ask her why she could do it so well at home and not in the pool. She looked at me and simply said, "The pool has a deep end."

Well, that didn't deter me and I continued explaining that she is roped off in the shallow end, far away from the deep end and should have no fears of it. Her irrational simple reply came again, "But I can see the deep end."

Many times in our struggles in this world, we are in the "shallow" end of our suffering, but in fear of seeing the "deep end" of death or increased suffering, we panic and freeze. We end up wallowing in the fear of "seeing the deep end".

As I clamored out of the Valley of the Shadow of Death, I realized what the depths of that pit were to me. God showed me that I had quite a few unnecessary and irrational fears of the deep end for which I needed to let go.

Once I released them, I learned an intimacy with our Lord that I had never felt or known before. He taught me some of His incredible attributes that filled the holes in my soul and became salve in my wounds. Let them work for you as well. Our God is a multi-tasking genius. The commander CEO has no hesitation with dispensation of compassion or comfort, or both simultaneously. The teacher functions easily as an intimate friend. He delights to be all to us in every moment of our day.

In "Land Between" by Jeff Manion the author points out that just as Israel had to be transformed from a people of slavery to a chosen people of God, I have to be transformed from selfish to selfless and from ungrateful to grateful. That kind of transformation doesn't happen over coffee. It happens over something jarring, like living in the desert for 40 years - or contracting chronic Lyme.

God led Israel through life threatening situations to prove HE can be trusted.

But remember what happened in the desert during those forty years; pillar of smoke by day and fire by night, manna and the quail. Every problem they had, every whine, every complaint, God was there ever-present saying to them "I can be trusted, I am able."

Look at your circumstances. Where are you and what complaints do you have? Is he listening? Is God responding? He is able.

The psalmist says "Relent Lord, how long will it be? Have compassion on your servants. Satisfy us in the morning with your unfailing love, that we man sing for joy and be glad all our days. Make us glad for as many days as you have afflicted us, for as many years as we have seen trouble" (Psalm 90:13-15). The same soul laments in Psalm 6:2-3 says "Have mercy on me Lord for I am faint; heal me Lord for my bones are in agony. My soul is in deep anguish. How long Lord, how long?"

No one knows how long your valley will last, when the end to your suffering will come or how deep your need for comfort has become, but He does. "Ah, Sovereign Lord, you have made the heavens and the earth by your great power and outstretched arm. Nothing is too hard for you" (Jeremiah 32:17). By verse 27, God himself speaks to Jeremiah saying, "I am the Lord, the God of all mankind. Is anything too hard for me?"

He is the end-all, the big kahuna, He is in this for you. He has power over it. He can heal it; He can sustain you if it's not healed. By His own personal admission, He has no limits and nothing is too hard for Him. I love how he says it to Moses "Is the Lord's arm too short? Now you will see whether or not what I say will come true for you" (Numbers 11:23). Healing Lyme remains within His reach for all time.

Hear it and believe it. What you have on your plate He can hold. He can hold it and do the dishes and clean up the kitchen at the same time and make sure the kids are ready for bed. He can hold it and mow the lawn and make sure your bills are paid and the mortgage doesn't default. He can hold it and keep your business running in your absence and step in as provider of the household. He can hold it and pay all your medical expenses. He can hold it. He is able.

Job responded to the Lord "I know that you can do all things; no purpose of yours can be thwarted. You asked, 'who is this that obscures my plans without knowledge' Surely I spoke of things I did not understand, things too wonderful for me to know" (Job 42:1-3)

God tells King Johoshaphat "Do not be afraid of discouraged because of this vast army. For the battle is not yours, but God's" (2 Chronicles 20:15).

The illness, this valley, this Lyme, this battle – the war in every cell of your body is not yours, but the Lord's. He is able.

"My flesh and my heart my fail, but God is the strength of my heart and my portion forever." (Psalm 73:26) Lord, give me the strength. He is able.

"Cast your cares on the Lord and he will sustain you; he will never let the righteous be shaken." (Psalm 55:22) Lord, sustain me through my weakness. He is able.

"Praise be to the Lord, to God our Savior, who daily bears our burdens." (Psalm 68:19) Lord, thank you for sharing my load. He is able.

"Cast all your anxiety of him because he cares for you." (1 Peter 5:7) Lord, remove my anxious reactions to the deep end. He is able.

"Come to me, all you who are weary and burdened, and I will give you rest. Take my yoke upon you and learn from me, for I am gentle and humble in heart, and you will find rest for your souls." (Matthew 11:28-29) Thank you Lord that I can find rest in you even when my physical body cannot find rest. He is able

Mark Batterson in "The Circle Maker" says "When you live by faith it often feels like you are risking your reputation. You are not. You are risking God's reputation. It's not your faith that is on the line, it's his faithfulness. Why? Because it's God who makes the promise, He is the only one who can keep it. The battle doesn't belong to you it belongs to God…it's about giving God an opportunity to prove himself to you." And sometimes even through you.

God can be trusted and he is able.

### Journal Entry:
*As you get older, you can relate to this phenomenon more – looking at yourself in the mirror and wondering who is looking back at you. It shocked me often when I saw my reflection when I was pregnant or holding a baby – I would think who is this mom? I didn't yet have an emotional attachment to that identity in myself, so it didn't seem like me at all.*

*Now chronically ill, I am shocked by what I see in my reflection. I see life escaping and devoid in my own eyes – in my own reflection that stares back at me, and it haunts me.*

*Disturbs me that my kids could see that, I can try to smile and make breakfast and peel myself off the couch, but they can see the evidence in my eyes. How could I stop this leak of life that seemed to seep out those empty eyes? Could God restore life to my eyes, let alone to my fading body? I am still in here. I can't see myself anymore, I look so dead.*

*I truly believe that the eyes are the window to the soul and that is why people who are sick look so dull and lifeless and how nurses with experience can just tell when people are on the edge of death. The eyes become listless and gone. I see this in myself and don't want to believe I was this far gone, this close to death.*

*But the eyes do not lie. I feel as though my soul itself was being reduced like a tire leaking air with no way to plug the hole. As my soul was escaping, it was taking more and more of my physical self with it. A giant migration was happening within my body cells – had they not gotten the memo that I was going to make it, I was going to survive this?*

*As I went from 115 to 105 to 95 then to 85 lbs., how much more of my soul was there left to leak out before my physical self gives way and departure is inevitable?*

Even as I began to heal, my physical body still felt and looked like a fragile withered flower. My clothes still hung off me and I had to cinch all my pants up with a belt or roll them down. I refused to buy a new wardrobe, but did purchase some new jeans at GoodWill that fit better. I haven't outgrown them all, but I did get rid of my first pair of skinny pants after I passed the 100 lb mark. Though strange to celebrate, find your own remarkable benchmarks to rejoice in. Share them with close friends and don't let them pass unnoticed.

As you celebrate your ascent from Lyme by honoring marks of personal achievement – no matter how small – don't be surprised that your focus shifts away from that ominous deep end of the pool. And when you are riding the waves of a good moment, you aren't fixated on the depth of the pool.

# 17

## Building Soldiers for Battle

*We have been called to heal wounds, to unite what has fallen apart, and to bring home those who have lost their way.*
*- St. Francis of Assisi*

On 9/11 I was in New York and worked 2 blocks from the World Trade Center. My commute involved taking the Path train into the subbasement of the WTC every morning from Hoboken, NJ. I had never experienced fear like that before. A soldier built for a battlefield of this kind of terror I am not. One thing I can tell you though was, when the fighter jets scrambled overhead within minutes, it came like reassurance that someone had my back. I was not down there alone in battle. The army has been called. On alert the soldiers are on their way. Someone is on this.

True comfort comes in knowing that God commands legions of warrior angels. He can speak it and bring it to pass. Fear not. The jets have been scrambled on your behalf. Your personal truth towers are under attack – your physical being and your spiritual self God is on this, He is powerful.

Recently in a bible study group discussion over the book "Beautiful Outlaw" by John Eldridge, we were discussing the chapter about the fierceness of Jesus. My friend Lisha, said so poignantly "I love this part. I don't know if it's me as a woman or just a person. I love seeing His power, His strength, to know He can rescue me and will do so with a drawn sword if necessary. I really needed to feel that today. It makes me feel so safe."

This reminds me of the conviction of Shadrach, Meshach and Abednego in refusing to bow down to the king's idol in Daniel chapter 3. They knew their God could rescue them, they knew his power AND his ability to choose not rescue them as well. "If we are thrown into the blazing furnace, the God we serve is able to deliver us from it, and he will deliver us from Your Majesty's hand. But even if he does not, we want you to know, Your Majesty that we will not serve your gods or worship the image of gold you have set up." (Daniel 3:16-18)

The three just believed that God could spring the rescue and that faith sustained them. Of course, we know He also carried out the rescue. But first they chose to believe in His fierceness. God had their backs and their fronts – a complete 360 degree shield.

God has the power to rescue; He has the power of divinity to know what is best for me at this moment and how long the fiery furnace will last. Even if He does not rescue right now, I need to stand firm. Even if the illness doesn't relent will you still believe He can heal it? Even if the pain doesn't go away will you have faith that He has power over it?

Our perspective from the weakness of a valley can view his power displayed in others' lives and make us wonder where His power in this illness is, my illness. Where is God's power in my weakness, where is my miracle of rising strength?

First and foremost, His power is displayed to glorify His kingdom, not remove obstacles so I can further my own kingdom here on earth. His power, His will, His choosing. But because of Christ, I have the opportunity to have that power living in me. When I accept Christ in my life, I get the Holy Spirit that indwells me.

"And his incomparably great power for us who believe. That power is the same as the mighty strength he exerted when he raised Christ from the dead and seated him at his right hand in the heavenly realms"(Eph 1:19-20). That power resides in me. His power exists in all who believes. The same power that raised Jesus from the dead and conquered Hades and resurrected and seated at the right hand of God – that power. That power remains in me. Not a little bit of it, not a smidge, not a drop, that whole power is given and living active in me.

Francis Chan says in his book the "Forgotten God" "if we today acted in the Holy Spirit's power the way the early church after Pentecost did, our churches of faith would be more active more vibrant, more powerful." That power is in me. He suggests reading the book of Acts. Let me encourage you to - get ready to have your socks blown off! That power is in me in this valley.

I don't just have access to the best; I have the best in me.

"Now to him who is able to do immeasurably more than all we ask or imagine, according to his power that is at work within us," (Eph 1:21). I don't know about you, but in this valley I can imagine many things, many options. I can picture not being sick, not being needy, I can remember not being like this. I can imagine and because I can imagine, I can ask. His power is at work within us and he can do MORE than all we ask or imagine. More. More than we ask or imagine. How would that feel? Incredible! Fabulous!

Mark Batterson in "The Circle Maker" says of prayer "unasked prayers are unanswered prayers." We might not ever know why some prayers go unanswered this side of heaven, but you can be sure of one thing. All the unasked prayers are a NO go. Given that – you must ask him. Ask him.

"I have been crucified with Christ and I no longer live, but Christ lives in me. The life I now live in the body, I live by faith in the son of God, who loved me and gave himself for me." (Galatians 2:20) Feel the abandonment of self? Feel the rescue?

He is our shield, our protector, our all powerful. "Trust in the Lord forever, for the Lord, the Lord himself, is the Rock eternal." (Isaiah 26:3-4) Sense who has your back and how fully you are covered.

My Bible study group just finished up Beth Moore's study of the book of James. I took such wisdom from the reminder of Elijah's actions from 1 Kings 18:41-46. James says of Elijah in verse 17 "Elijah was man just like us. He prayed earnestly that it would not rain, and it did not rain on the land for three and a half years. Again he prayed, and the heavens gave rain, and the earth produced its crops."

I know what waiting for rain feels like. Do you? How long has your drought lasted? How long have you prayed in earnest and waited? But read about Elijah's perseverance and

136

faithfulness in I Kings 18. "But Elijah climbed to the top of Carmel, bent down to the ground and put his face between his knees. 'Go and look toward the sea,' he told his servant. And he went up and looked. 'There is nothing there,' he said. Seven times Elijah said, 'Go back.' The seventh time the servant reported, 'A cloud as small as a man's hand is rising from the sea.' So Elijah said, 'Go...'" His rescue came life a frog-chocking gullywasher- unmistakably God

Knowing God deeply gave Elijah the courage to not give up. Why not? He recognized the character of the God he served. He knew his God was powerful, he knew his God was faithful and he was certain that if he stayed prostrate in reverence and in awe of that power long enough, the answer would come. Even more amazing to me, is that the "answer" to the prayer would have been the rain itself, but not to Elijah. All he needed to see on the horizon is a fist-sized cloud. A fist-sized cloud on the horizon is not a rain storm and in my opinion, not an answer to prayer. But Elijah recognized God's work and he knew of His power and His faithfulness. That it went from wisp to washout speaks of God's ability to deluge drought in His power.

Don't give up hope; don't give up on God's power. Your fist-sized cloud could already be there on the horizon – it's just not raining yet. But it will arrive. He has heard, He is powerful and He is listening. Ask. Wait. And look up in confidence.

My mentor and heart-friend Rose, is a walking 83 year-young evangelist. Only in the heart of Rose Marie did God plant such tenacity and boldness to share His kingdom. Upon her dear

137

husband's death after 56 years of marriage, she witnessed to one of the EMT's that came in the ambulance to get her dead husband's body.

At a recent retreat, she encouraged a young vibrant worker behind the breakfast counter who was singing to give it a good 'hallelujah'. I heard the chorus ring out across the room to see if indeed my instincts were right – Rose Marie had just been there beside him. How did I know? Because I know her. I spend time with her and know her character and how she will react. It spills out of her like a breadcrumb trail behind a toddler eating cookies.

Do you know God this well? Do I know God like I know my Rose Marie? I need to. I desperately need to know Him this well, so I can trust Him and so the roots on my faith can grow deeper and deeper.

The day after 9/11, I was gathering with my discipleship group from church and one of the ladies got out her Bible and read "Whoever dwells in the shelter of the Most High will rest in the shadow of the Almighty. I will say of the Lord, He is my refuge and my fortress, my God in whom I trust. Surely he will save you from the fowler's snare and from the deadly pestilence. He will cover you with his feathers, and under his wings you will find refuge; his faithfulness will be your shield and rampart. You will not fear the terror of night, nor the arrow that flies by day, nor the pestilence that talks in the darkness nor the plague that destroys at midday. A thousand may fall at your side, ten thousand at your right hand, but it will not come near you."

(from Psalm 91:1) Do you see the ominous date of the terrorist strike encoded in this reference?

Don't fear the terror that plagues you at night or in the day in this valley. He will surely save you and cover you. In Him you will find refuge. His faithfulness is your shield. His reputation in faithfulness is on the line, remember.

*"Those who know your name trust in you, for you, Lord, have never forsaken those who seek you." (Psalm 9:10)*

*"I know you can do all things; no purpose of yours can be thwarted." (Job 42:2)*

*"The righteous person may have many troubles, but the Lord delivers him from them all." (Psalm 34:19)*

*"The Lord makes firm the steps of the one who delights in him; though he may stumble, he will not fall for the Lord upholds him with his hand." (Psalm 37:23-24)*

*"I will rescue him; I will protect him, for he acknowledges my name. He will call on me and I will answer him, I will be with him in trouble, I will deliver him and honor him." (Psalm 91:14-15a)*

God is powerful, He is mighty to save you.


*Journal of a fellow Lyme sufferer:*

*Are you sick? In order to heal, you have to be ready for it. Are you ready? I am. I am no longer a victim. I am no longer angry. One day you will look back and it will all be a valuable lesson learned. I know those of you deeply in the throes of disease won't understand what I am trying to say or may even be offended by what I am saying. If you are offended you probably need to dig deeper and ask yourself some important questions. But one day you will wake up in the morning and it will hit you like an "aha moment" and you will see what I mean. Then you will start on your path to wellness.*

*You have to KNOW that you will get better. That within the next few minutes you will feel a little bit better than you do right now. Know it with every part of your being and forgive yourself when you doubt it. When someone tells you that this will be a long hard battle, stick your nose in the air and tell them where to stick it because it won't be for you.*

Though you may not have chosen it, this Lyme is your battle ground where you will be tested beyond your wills and abilities. You have faced and are facing an extreme terror of indescribable proportion. Now, rise up as a soldier ready for battle – geared up, sword in hand, outfitted with the whole armor of God.

# 18

## This is for Me?

*...We will stand amazed to see the topside of the tapestry and how God beautifully embroidered each circumstance into a pattern for our good and His glory.*
*- Joni Eareckson Tada*

When my son was in kindergarten, his class was assigned the chapel performance at his Christian school. They opted for a theatrical interpretation of Genesis one, since they had been studying the creation. Each time one of the children read about a part of his creation, all the kids joined in chorus and echoed it was "goooooooo-ooood" adding about three syllables to the word for emphasis. The effect was memorable. If you are from the south, you completely understand, because we always add to one syllable words for "hickness" and emphasis. In your mind, you can hear it, it sounds like Jeff Foxworthy. Everything God made was "goooo-ooood."

*"God saw all that he had made, and it was very good."* *(Genesis 1:31)*

*"God created mankind in his own image, in the image of God he created them; male and female he created them."* *(Genesis 1:27)*

*"Everyone who is called by my name, whom I created for my glory, whom I formed and made."* *(Isaiah 43:7)*

He made you and me this way. He made you goooo-ooood. Very goooo-ooood. He made each of us, each element of His

141

creation gooooo-ooood. There are no mistakes. Yes, it is a fallen world and when sin entered the garden our earthly bodies changed and became broken. The earth changed and became broken. But the scripture reminds us that He still is the Creator, the one who takes and gives life.

*"For you created my inmost being; you knit me together in my mother's womb. I praise you because I am fearfully and wonderfully made. Your works are wonderful and I know that full well. My frame was not hidden from you when I was made in the secret place, when I was woven together in the depths of the earth. Your eyes saw my unformed body; all the days ordained for me were written in your book before one of them came to be." (Psalm 139:13-16)*

He knit me together in my mother's womb; the weak parts, strong parts, the parts that would be stricken with Lyme, the conditions that would allow it to attack. Now follow me here, because there are mothers out there who can understand this. He knit my children together in my Lyme-infested womb. And when He did it, the scripture assures us they were fearfully and wonderfully made.

It is easier to understand that He chose this journey for me. But for my kids? For them? For them. He chose this and knit them together and allowed the Lyme attack for them too. Pain above pain to see them suffer. Guilt upon guilt to believe I could have housed this illness and passed it unknowingly to them. But read it again and receive it in as truth.

My frame, my illness, my disease was neither hidden from Him when I was made, nor when my kids were made in the secret place. All these days were ordained for me and for them,

142

written in His book before even one of them came to be. The end was already determined before my Lyme exploded. Before I got sick, in the book I was already well. Before the kids were a glimmer in my husband's eye, they already had Lyme and then were healed.

Hear that truth and take it to heart. There are only two ways this illness can end for you. Both are so brilliant and amazing. The one chosen for you is already written in the book of life in the throne room of heaven. You will be healed and you will get better and you will survive. Or God will choose this to be your time and you will be ushered into his presence, pain and suffering-free. These are the two options. Here or Eternity. Glory upon glory, even in being here in our lack of health we still get the promise of eternity too.

I don't take lightly when I say only two options, because I realize in our earthly timeline both could include suffering until that end. That suffering, as we've discussed, explodes and overtakes our lives and all those around us. It is intense. It is huge. It is a beast.

Knowing that there is an end to it, could you endure it one more day? Or make it through by leaning on God one day at a time? If we can grasp the truth that God is able, He is powerful and He created us, then does that yield itself to endurance?

Imagine being pain-free and focus your eyes on eternity. Read about heaven (See Resources section for uplifting book titles). Our life here is only a breath. The days are long and the years are short. Hold fast to this and trust in the One who is Faithful and True.

*"See now that I myself am he! There is no God besides me. I put to death and I bring to life, I have wounded and I will heal, and no one can deliver out of my hand." (Deuteronomy 32:39) He decides. He already decided. He gives breath. He gives life. "From the dust of the ground and breathed into his nostrils the breath of life, and the man became a living being." (Genesis 2:7)*

*"The Lord gives and the Lord takes away. Blessed be the name of the Lord." (Job 1:21)*

### Journal Entry:

*I meditate on Psalm 27:13-14 as a prayer mantra through this valley. It's the promise I cling to, the message He told me was mine. So what does take heart mean? As I research and look up "take heart", it seems to mean the Lord is asking me to remember. But why doesn't He use the word remember then? I think taking heart is more than remembering – it is more like a tattoo or searing a brand of His promises into our hearts and faith. He wants me to take these promises and brand them permanently into my heart. A brand cannot fade, his promises transcend time, and they will not fade. He does not change and does not fail.*

*The overflow of hope comes from the Holy Spirit using those "brands" on my heart and promises of God himself in the overflow of my life. What a revelation, so simple but so profound to me. I thought I had been through valleys in which my faith and outlook had been clarified, but this valley has been like a corrective Lasik surgery to my faith.*

*As I climb back uphill again out of a pit, I ask Him, "how long must I suffer for your sake to achieve glory for your name?"*

I continue to pray for each Lyme sufferer that this valley will transform your faith and your life. I pray that Lyme disease and all of its ugly, exhausting fear and pain will result in true meaning for you and your family. And when you ask "this is for me?" you will truly understand why.

# 19

## Nothing is Hidden

*Worrying is carrying tomorrow's load with today's strength-carrying two days at once. It is moving into tomorrow ahead of time. Worrying doesn't empty tomorrow of its sorrow, it empties today of its strength.*
*- Corrie ten Boom*

In my twenties, I was in complete rebellion against the world, my parents, and most importantly, the Lord. I was an art student and was all over the place, Chicago, London, New York. I had many bad experiences and traumas that I knew made me stronger, but in my rebellion. I couldn't see God anywhere. How could He let these things happen? It seemed to strengthen my resolve that He was nowhere to be seen. He held His silence. All further proof that I didn't need Him to exist.

Years later, after I came back to faith and to my senses, I travelled back to London for a business trip. I was so excited. I hadn't been back since I had spent two rebellious semesters there during college. An art major, I had spent many, many hours in the museums of London on my own studying and with professors in class. I couldn't wait to get back to my favorite of these museums, the National Gallery off Trafalgar Square.

*"Nothing in all creation is hidden from God's sight. Everything is uncovered and lay bare before the eyes of him to whom we must give account." (Hebrews 4:12-13)*

I spent an entire semester in the Renaissance wing and I fell in love with that era. So immediately checked into the hotel, and forgetting my jetlag, jumped in the first cabbie to the National Gallery and went off to admire my favorite pieces. I stopped at the first one and immediately began to cry, the second generated more tears. I hurried back to the gift shop to purchase pen and paper so I could write down what I was transpiring inside.

The first painting depicted John the Baptist baptizing Jesus with the Holy Spirit descending as a dove (Piero della Francesca, The Baptism of Christ). The second represented Jesus washing the disciple's feet in the Upper Room (Tintoretto – Christ washing the disciple's feet). On and on it went for me that day of memorable return. Jesus lived in every room, His life story retold through the Renaissance painters. I had stood there and admired the art on my original encounters and completely missed the artist. Jesus himself.

How could I have doubted that God was there in my rebellion waiting and watching - and I would dare say - protecting? God of the universe was there and I missed Him all those years ago. Now I was literally weeping in the museum room after room His Spirit awakened in me and testifying to Him in my tears.

"For the eyes of the Lord range throughout the earth to strengthen those whose hearts are fully committed to him." (2 Chronicles 16:9) I knew from being raised in a church that "God sees all things". But in rebellion and separating myself from His presence, I thought I could go somewhere, hurt and rebel and He would not be there.

What a glorious promise is inferred here. What if His eyes roam the earth looking and waiting for more to become believers to enable them to become fully committed to Him? Didn't He do that to me throughout my rebellious period? He didn't just roam the earth looking, He placed himself there. Look around you and look backward. Ask Him to show you where He was and where He is. Be ready to be amazed, He is there. He has been there all along.

*"If you then though you are evil, know how to give good gifts to your children, how much more will your Father in heaven give good gifts to those who ask him!" (Matthew 7:11)*

God is standing at the ready. His eyes roam the earth waiting, watching and preparing opportunity. He is waiting at the ready to give us good gifts. "Every good and perfect gift is from above, coming down from the Father of heavenly lights, who does not change like shifting shadows." (James 1:17) "He who did not spare his own Son, but gave him up for us all – how will he not also, along with him, graciously give us all things?" (Romans 8:32)

He was there. He is there. God stands ready to give you good gifts. So what do we do with that if we are too weak to ask and to think? Oh, He is ready for that too. He is not just ready, willing, and able and everywhere we need him to be, he is our advocate, ready to speak on our behalf.

I knew the scripture well, "Let us approach God's throne of grace with confidence, so that we may receive mercy and find grace to help us in our time of need." (Hebrews 4:16 ) But in this season of illness, I had no confidence at times in anything – all I had was a great deal of the "time of need" part. Here's what we need to know: "We have this hope as an anchor for the soul, firm and secure. It enters the inner sanctuary behind the curtain, where our forerunner, Jesus has entered on our behalf." (Hebrews 6:19)

Jesus will do it on our behalf. And listen to this, Jesus also sent us a helper who intercedes for us also. "In the same way, the Spirit helps us in our weakness. We do not know what we ought to pray for, but the Spirit himself intercedes for us through wordless groans. And he who searches our hearts knows the mind of the Spirit, because the Spirit intercedes for God's people in accordance with the will of God." (Romans 8:26-27)

In my rebellious period, I made assumptions about God and about His activity in my life. But nothing in God's nature assumes. Luci Swindoll writes in Women of Faith devotional:

*"I am having computer problems today and it seems as if they will go on forever. It is like being broke and assuming I will never have money again, or sick and thinking I will never get well again, or discouraged and believing I will never be carefree again. But if I think like that for long, life isn't fun anymore. It feels too hard and I begin believing my erroneous judgment is more reliable than God's word. I forget that God is always at work on my behalf. The test in your life today is part of God's plan. You may not like it. You may want to throw in the towel. But God is using it to grow you up. Don't support for one minute he doesn't know what he is doing."*

The dictionary.com defines an advocate as: a person who pleads for in behalf or another, an intercessor. My favorite is how intercessor is defined: to act or interpose in behalf of someone in difficulty or trouble, as by pleading or petition.

God is in this thing. I am, and you are, in trouble and experiencing a difficult life. God uses both Jesus the son and the Holy Spirit to plead, petition on our behalf. The Holy Spirit is interceding for us in the throne room of heaven even now. Do you truly believe that? Do you have that confidence?

*Lymie, do you have a personal relationship with Jesus Christ? Do you feel assured that He is your advocate and that the Holy Spirit is dwelling in your heart available for giving you strength and encouragement in the face of this storm? If you have any doubts, please, right now, take a moment of quiet reflection and ask Jesus to come into your life. Be assured of your salvation in eternity and pray this simple prayer:*

*Lord, I am a sinner and know that only through the saving work of Jesus dying on the cross that my sins were paid for. I accept Jesus's act of sacrifice on my behalf and ask Him right now to come into my life as my personal Lord and Savior so I can be assured of spending my eternity with you and the rest of this earthly life with the Holy Spirit dwelling in my heart providing the strength I need to endure. In Jesus Name Amen.*

Heed the spiritual call amid the physical weakness of Lyme disease. All who seek God will find Him. Then you won't stroll by the masterful artwork of life and miss the life-changing subject matter. Nothing is hidden. Let God reveal himself in your life today.

# 20

## The After-Party: Post Lyme Syndrome

*God reveals himself in rearview mirrors.*
*- Ann Voskamp*

Post Lyme Syndrome is not a phrase you will hear many doctors talk about and certainly you can't even find much under a Google search, but ask any Lymie and you know that it exists.

I have heard described to me what happens to an amputee patient after the trauma. They still have pain in the missing appendage. Phantom pain. How is it that the brain and nerves register pain in something that is not there anymore? Memory. Your brain is not the only place that stores memories. Each cell in your body stores memories - cell memory.

Post Lyme Syndrome has many facets, and one is cell memory. For months (and even still today) after I had no ammonia in my body, no trace of the active spirochete called Lyme, I would have the same symptoms at various times, after painting the kitchen cabinets, after walking three days in a row, before my menstrual cycle would begin.

Why on earth would my body register Lyme symptoms instead of tired muscles? Lyme symptoms instead of menstrual cramps? The answer lies in cell memory.

When the body has been in a chronic health state, all the last settings were on "panic" or "all hands on deck". Initially, when the body needs to react to something, it calls up its last setting and registers it instead. So, if any severe emotional, spiritual or physical occurrence has happened, the body can misfire the symptoms.

To a vastly paranoid and uber sensitive Lymie, this tucks healing into a tailspin. You are getting better and have the natural setbacks at times, then you have these "false" setbacks also. Which ones are real? Unfortunately, it is difficult to tell the difference. One way to distinguish in some people, the "false" ones usually pass faster and don't keep going down. As a patient keeping a positive outlook and trying to look forward, you get to dangle on the edge of the cliff waiting to see if you topple over or get to walk back from the edge. Not appealing huh?

Good news, just like discerning what type of crying a new baby has – wet diaper, hunger, pain, or tired, a Lymie patient will get very good at reading her/his body. Listen and pay attention, journal it, talk to your doctor and talk to other Lyme patients. Every 12-18 months every cell in your body will have been regenerated, so the memories in those cells will be erased or rebooted like a computer to not misfire incorrect information.

Many small plane crashes are pilot error, either in not checking equipment/fuel levels properly or in not trusting their instruments. If a pilot is flying in IFR conditions (flying by the instruments because visual line of sight is blocked), then a pilot must trust his instruments. There is no horizon line, nothing to look out the windshield at and get your bearing, only instruments to trust. In an accident,a pilot will go down on gut instinct and not trusting the instruments.

In post Lyme the instincts of the body are still recovering from Lyme and they are also shrouded in fear and discouragement. The instruments of the body aren't registering the correct responses. Fake symptoms and fear will feed into each other and perpetuate another crash. This is what makes recovery so difficult and frustrating. There is only one truth to fly on and trust in and that's God's truth. God can help me discern what is a real symptom from a fake one, God can remove the fear from the cycle and help me not crash.

If you use the storm analogy for Lyme again, then every time it rains or the wind blows, the body acts like it's another tornado. It's basically like an overacting drama queen. The symptoms are real, but the readings are false.

Then there is the aftermath of a tornado.The path of destruction left behind the tornado has to be "fixed", rebuilt and restored. Have you ever driven through a tornado path after the storm? It is hard to find your way around with all the landmarks and road signs gone. Have you seen how everything is flattened? Then months later as you see it cleared, the stubble of trees look funny as leaves are growing off the stump, not the missing branches. Everything is healing and growing but still looks a bit off.

Your body after Lyme has experienced a path of destruction. Depending on where the Lyme attacked your liver, your intestines, your heart, your brain - all have to be rebuilt. Until

154

each organ is rebuilt, all the road signs for normal body function are missing, all the landmarks are destroyed.

Have you ever noticed when they interview people after the wake of a tornado coming and devastating their neighborhoods, they almost always focus on what they have, not what is gone? They are so thankful their family, or their neighbors, or their pets are alright. They will rebuild. Develop a thankful heart over the things that are working correctly post Lyme.

And what does rebuilding take even more than money? Time. Time and energy and flat out perseverance. No matter how much time, money and energy you have to give, when you rebuild after a tornado, the house won't be the same. The yard and the trees won't be the same. It will look different feel different. Some things might actually be better. Since Lyme builds slowly in most of us, there are many symptoms we had learned to live with which are finally gone upon its departure.

Also, the rebuilding does something for our care of the body. I will be much more cautious in the future about how much physical/emotional/spiritual stress I subject my body to at one time and for how long (within my control). Exercising and eating right are a no-brainer – we did that, but we will continue to even more. Sure I miss eating gluten and dairy and eating at some of my favorite restaurants, but in the grand scheme of things, I prefer to be physically strong and raise my kids. If the gluten and dairy put even a hint of physical risk for my body to fight off the Lyme or other co-infections, then it is not worth it.

God reminded me last year while studying the book of Revelation through Beth Moore's bible study that we get to feast in heaven. Feast, really feast on any food group and more delicious food than we can fathom. And none of it will cause a problem in our heavenly bodies, no bloating, no nausea, no cramping, no problems.

I am proud to be left standing after my storm came through. Proud to be standing amid the destruction and being allowed the opportunity to rebuild. I want more functioning, I want thriving vitality, I want a newly rebuilt structure that can withstand the next storm more soundly and boast of a renewed spirit that comes from a rebuilding season.

*Do you not know? Have you not heard?*
*The Lord is the everlasting God, the Creator of the ends of the earth.*
*He will not grow tired or weary, and his understanding no one can fathom.*
*He gives strength to the weary and increases the power of the weak.*
*Even youths grow tired and weary, and young men stumble and fall;*
*but those who hope in the Lord will renew their strength.*
*They will soar on wings like eagles; they will run and not grow weary, they will walk and not be faint. (Isaiah 38:17-20)*

The old saying goes that you have to crawl before you walk. The Lord says it right here, you have to walk and not be faint and run and not grow weary and then soar. Soar. The Lord will never grow tired and there is no end to his strength for us. The reservoir is always full. There is no bottom, no end.

We are in a serious drought in Kansas this year, even with the surprising 21 inches of snow we got dumped on us; we are still 20 inches behind in rainfall. I have no idea how they know that, but I can drive by the river and see how low it is. I can see photos on the news of the local reservoir and see how there is not much water left. Boat docks sit dry by its edge, reminding me how limited earth's natural resources are.

God's well never runs dry. It is never empty.

After seeing a commercial pretending to be old-fashioned black and white TV, my spiritual life shift seems a little like that. Going from the sound and picture quality of an old black and white TV to a new high definition. flat screen with surround sound. Before Lyme, I thought I was walking with the Lord, trusting Him, loving Him and serving Him. Then the storm hit and I realized that the black and white TV faith was not going to cut it in the storm. Putting my faith to the test in this storm drew me to the Lord for an anchor. I needed more and wanted more and knew Him better. I know Him better. Now my faith shines in high def.

I loved growing up and watching Cubs baseball on my Papa's black and white TV. I loved it because he loved it and I loved being with him. The games were exciting and I could tell what was going on and who was winning. But to watch baseball on a high def. flat screen, there is no comparison. Post Lyme heightens not only our physical senses but our spiritual senses as well.

*Journal Entry:*

*Think back to 16 years old and driving for the first time. Remember feeling so weird being alone on your own thinking "I can't believe they are trusting me to do this." Feeling guilty somehow because it didn't seem comfortable or right just yet to be on your own in the car. Or going off to college the first time or voting or ordering your first beer – wearing that responsibility the first time was like putting on a stiff jacket or new pair of shoes, noticeably new and feeling odd until they get worn in, like pretending to play grownup.*

*Sometimes that's how I feel lately. Driving alone in the car by myself or with the kids after 15-16 months of always being chauffeured or chaperoned, feels like I'm doing something wrong or trying to get away with something. Am I really old enough, safe enough and responsible enough to be doing this by myself?*

*Yesterday I was keenly aware of this as I was driving another friend's daughter to school. I was gripping at 10 and 2 white-knuckled, thinking am I trustworthy to be having this responsibility?*

*I had to pray the whole time to keep the panic cloud from smothering me whole. It's as if 24 years of driving has been erased completely from my memory banks. I remember being strong and responsible at some point. I know I used to be that person, but somehow it feels like that memory has faded and is barely recognizable.*

More time has passed since I had to find my footing post Lyme. I find it more frustrating when I begin to slip into my old ways instead of find my new ones. I accept and embrace the new me after Lyme because my life perspective has grown richer. My viewpoint possesses one of eternal things, not temporal ones. I don't want to lose this distilled person, this higher foothold for anything. I want relationships to be more important than what is on TV each night. I want my kid's spiritual future and worldview to take precedence over what's happening on Facebook.

I don't want life to get out of balance again. Allow Post Lyme to serve as the rearview mirror that provides you higher definition for your perspective. Not everyone gets such visual aid, so make it count.

# 21

## Claim a Promise

*So is my word that goes out from my mouth: It will not return to
me empty, but will accomplish what I desire and achieve the purpose
for which I sent it.
Isaiah 55:11*

It is from this verse in Isaiah that this chapter is written. In the valley I have found it bountiful to claim a promise in His word that relates to the struggles I am personally having, whether health- related or spiritual or both. God promises that His word will not return to Him empty, but will accomplish what He desires and achieve the purpose for which He sent it. There is no way to actually know God's purpose, except by the power and discernment of the Holy Spirit working through us. Pray about it, search the scriptures and find your own or look through the scriptures in this chapter.

I have the scripture promise that God laid upon my heart right in the middle of the crash and it written on a tattered and torn paper still tucked in my devotional book and I claim it still:

*I remain confident of this: I will see the goodness of the Lord in the land of the living. Wait for the Lord; be strong and take heart and wait for the Lord. (Psalm 27:13-14)*

I also have prayed and chanted often in the bad pain days: The Lord replied, My presence will go with you and I will give you rest. (Exodus 33:14)

Over my kids I have claimed: The bolts of your gates will be iron and bronze, and your strength will equal your days. (Deuteronomy 33:25)

*See now that I myself am he! There is no god besides me. I put to death and I bring to life, I have wounded and I will heal, and no one can deliver out of my hand. (Deuteronomy 32:39)*

My fellow patient and friend Caity has claimed this promise: Look at the nations and watch— and be utterly amazed. For I am going to do something in your days that you would not believe, even if you were told. (Habakkuk 1:5)

Look to these scripture promises and hold fast to them as an anchor to help you weather this storm. His word will not return to Him empty. I couldn't possibly, no matter how long I deliberated, think of the proper and perfect words to leave you with. This journey, this valley in all its intensity, is not for the faint of heart. You need more than my encouragement and my story of hope to arrive at the end of yours.

As this book closes, all I can do is to leave you with words that contain everlasting hope. Words that house a staying power not found on earth. Words that can penetrate pain, exhaustion, depression and loss. Use these scripture promises as something to anchor to in your "perfect storm". They will not let you down.

I pray for you, I am praying for you as you journey out of your Lyme pit. Find hope and incremental joy each day where you can. Grasp your open windows with vigor and live them to the fullest. I will rejoice with you on your mountaintop of healing.

## Claim a Promise

Though you have made me see troubles through this Lyme disease, many and bitter, you will restore my life again, from the depths of this illness, you will again bring me up. You will increase my honor and comfort me once more.

*Though you have made me see troubles, many and bitter, you will restore my life again; from the depths of the earth you will again bring me up. You will increase my honor and comfort me once more. (Psalm 71:20-21)*

I will not fear, for the Lord has redeemed me and summoned me by name. When I pass through the waters, He will be with me; and will I pass through the rivers, they will not sweep over me. When I walk through this Lyme fire, I will not be burned; the flames of this illness will not set me ablaze. For the Lord is my God, the Holy One of Israel, My Savior. Since I am precious and honored in His sight and because He loves me, I do not have to be afraid.

*But now, this is what the Lord says—he who created you, Jacob, he who formed you, Israel: "Do not fear, for I have redeemed you; I have summoned you by name; you are mine. When you pass through the waters, I will be with you; and when you pass through the rivers, they will not sweep over you. When you walk through the fire, you will not be burned; the flames will not set you ablaze. For I am the Lord your God, the Holy One of Israel, your Savior; I give Egypt for your ransom, Cush[a] and Seba in your stead. Since you are precious and honored in my sight, and because I love you, I will give people in exchange for you, nations in exchange for your life. Do not be afraid, for I am with you; I will bring your children from the east and gather you from the west. (Isaiah 43:1-5)*

The Lord Jesus will bind up my broken heart, he will give me freedom from this Lyme captivity and release me from its darkness. He will comfort me when I mourn and provide for my every need. He will show me how to praise Him in the illness and take away my despair. Then I will be called an oak of righteousness, a planting of the Lord for the display of His splendor. Holy Spirit help rebuild the ruins this disease has taken on my physical, emotional and spiritual self and restore it to your creation, fearfully and wonderfully made. Instead of shame I will receive a double portion and rejoice. Everlasting joy will be mine.

*He has sent me to bind up the brokenhearted, to proclaim freedom for the captives and release from darkness for the prisoners, to proclaim the year of the Lord's favor and the day of vengeance of our God, to comfort all who mourn, and provide for those who grieve in Zion—to bestow on them a crown of beauty instead of ashes, the oil of joy instead of mourning, and a garment of praise instead of a spirit of despair. They will be called oaks of righteousness, a planting of the Lord for the display of his splendor. They will rebuild the ancient ruins and restore the places long devastated; Instead of your shame you will receive a double portion, and instead of disgrace you will rejoice in your inheritance. And so you will inherit a double portion in your land, and everlasting joy will be yours. (Isaiah 61: 1-4, 7, Psalm 139:13-14)*

Because the Sovereign Lord helps me, I will not be disgraced in this Lyme disease.

Therefore have I set my face like flint to the disease, and I know I will not be put to shame.

*Because the Sovereign Lord helps me, I will not be disgraced.*

*Therefore have I set my face like flint, and I know I will not be put to shame. (Isaiah 50:7)*

I know you are using this Lyme disease to discipline me for my good that I may share in your holiness.Despite the pain I trust in you. I know that later this pain and illness will produce a harvest of righteousness and peace for me and that it will train me to be a better mom, wife, friend, grandmother, servant, believer.

*They disciplined us for a little while as they thought best; but God disciplines us for our good, in order that we may share in his holiness. No discipline seems pleasant at the time, but painful. Later on, however, it produces a harvest of righteousness and peace for those who have been trained by it. (Hebrews 12:10-11)*

Lord, you have made the heavens and the earth and this Lyme disease by your great power and outstretched arm. Nothing is too hard for you, including this illness in me.

*Ah, Sovereign Lord, you have made the heavens and the earth by your great power and outstretched arm. Nothing is too hard for you. (Jeremiah 32:17)*
*I am the Lord, the God of all mankind. Is anything too hard for me? (Jeremiah 32:27)*

Thank you that you know the plans for my life, plans to prosper me and not to harm me through this Lyme disease, plans to give me a hope and a future.

*For I know the plans I have for you," declares the Lord, "plans to prosper you and not to harm you, plans to give you hope and a future. (Jeremiah 29:11)*

Thank you that you alone know the number of my days and the length of my suffering and that you see fit to use this for my good. I trust you as the God who gives life to the dead and calls into being things that were not.

*As it is written: "I have made you a father of many nations." He is our father in the sight of God, in whom he believed—the God who gives life to the dead and calls into being things that were not. (Romans 4:17)*

*And we know in all things, God works to the good of those who love Him who have been called according to His purpose. (Romans 8:28)*

Lord please bestow upon me the wisdom of how to traverse this illness. Give me the next steps to healing and guide me to the right doctor and treatment that you have chosen for me. Open doors of opportunity for me that no man can close.

*If any of you lacks wisdom, you should ask God, who gives generously to all without finding fault, and it will be given to you. (James 1:5)*

*I know your deeds. See, I have placed before you an open door that no one can shut. I know that you have little strength, yet you have kept my word and have not denied my name. (Revelation 3:8)*

I will look to the Lord and His strength and I will seek His face always even in this illness.

*Look to the Lord and his strength; seek his face always. (1 Chronicles 16:11)*

I am from God and I can overcome this Lyme disease, because the one who is in me is greater than the one who is in the world and in this illness.

*You, dear children, are from God and have overcome them, because the one who is in you is greater than the one who is in the world. (1 John 4:4)*

Lord help me triumph over this illness by the power of the risen Savior Jesus Christ. Let me use my testimony through Lyme to glorify your kingdom. Help me to speak of your faithfulness and provision through this storm of life and not be afraid of death.

*They triumphed over him by the blood of the Lamb and by the word of their testimony; they did not love their lives so much as to shrink from death. (Revelation 12:11)*

It is from this dark place that I have been able to see and know you more. Continue to reveal your strength and power and light to me in this dark place. Use this circumstance to increase my joy in You and give me a heart that rejoices at all times. Give me contentment where you have placed me and meet my every need here in this place. Help me to not be anxious but pray with thanksgiving at all times. Send me your peace which will guard my heart and mind in Jesus.

*The people walking in darkness have seen a great light; on those living in the land of deep darkness a light has dawned. You have enlarged the nation and increased their joy; they rejoice before you as people rejoice at the harvest, as warriors rejoice when dividing the plunder. (Isaiah 9:2-3)*

*Rejoice in the Lord always. I will say it again: Rejoice! Let your gentleness be evident to all. The Lord is near. Do not be anxious about anything, but in every situation, by prayer and petition, with thanksgiving, present your requests to God. And the peace of God, which transcends all understanding, will guard your hearts and your minds in Christ Jesus. (Philippians 4:4-7)*

166

*I am not saying this because I am in need, for I have learned to be content whatever the circumstances. I know what it is to be in need, and I know what it is to have plenty. I have learned the secret of being content in any and every situation, whether well fed or hungry, whether living in plenty or in want. I can do all this through him who gives me strength. (Philippians 4:11-13)*

Thank you that, through this Lyme disease, you can keep me from stumbling and feeling sorry for myself and remove my pity parties. Walk me through this storm without fault and with great joy.

*To him who is able to keep you from stumbling and to present you before his glorious presence without fault and with great joy. (Jude 1:24)*

Lord, help me to continue living my life through this illness rooted and built up in You and strengthen my faith in it. Give me a heart and attitude of thankfulness and do not let me fall victim to the enemy and his use of this illness to destroy any part of my life, my relationships, my provision, my faith and my emotional self. Thank you that, in Jesus, I have been brought to fullness and he is the power and authority over everything, including this Lyme.

*So then, just as you received Christ Jesus as Lord, continue to live your lives in him, rooted and built up in him, strengthened in the faith as you were taught, and overflowing with thankfulness. See to it that no one takes you captive through hollow and deceptive philosophy, which depends on human tradition and the elemental spiritual forces of this world rather than on Christ. For in Christ all the fullness of the Deity lives in bodily form, and in Christ you have been brought to fullness. He is the head over every power and authority. (Colossians 2:6-10)*

167

The Lord is my shepherd, and I lack for nothing. He gives me rest and peace and refreshes my soul. He will guide me along the right paths for His name's sake. Even though I walk through the valley of the shadow of death, I will not fear for you are with me and you will comfort me. You prepare a celebration for me and anoint me with oil until my cup overflows. Surely your goodness and love will follow me all the days of my life and I will dwell in the house of the Lord forever.

*The Lord is my shepherd, I lack nothing. He makes me lie down in green pastures, he leads me beside quiet waters, he refreshes my soul.*

*He guides me along the right paths for his name's sake.*

*Even though I walk through the valley of the shadow of death, I will fear no evil, for you are with me; your rod and your staff, they comfort me.*

*You prepare a table before me in the presence of my enemies. You anoint my head with oil; my cup overflows.*

*Surely your goodness and love will follow me all the days of my life, and I will dwell in the house of the Lord forever. (Psalm 23)*


Lord, I have suffered much and I suffer still; preserve my life according to your word.

*I have suffered much; preserve my life, Lord, according to your word. (Psalm 119:107)*


Help me and give me strength my God, according to your promise that I will live. Keep my hope steadfast in you.

*Sustain me, my God, according to your promise, and I will live; do not let my hopes be dashed. (Psalm 119:116)*

It is not cause for shame why I am suffering as I am, because I know in Jesus Christ that I believe and I am convinced that He is able to guard what I have entrusted to Him each day.

*That is why I am suffering as I am. Yet this is no cause for shame, because I know whom I have believed, and am convinced that he is able to guard what I have entrusted to him until that day. (2 Timothy 1:12)*

Lord your plans will be and what you have purposed for my life will happen. Thank you that I can rest in this for my next minutes and my tomorrow.

*The Lord Almighty has sworn, "Surely, as I have planned, so it will be, and as I have purposed, so it will happen." (Isaiah 14:24)*

Surely it is for my benefit that I am suffering such anguish. In your love you keep me from the pit of destruction. You have put my sins behind your back. For the grave cannot praise you, death cannot sing your praise; The living, the living – they praise you, as I am doing today.

I will tell my children about your faithfulness. The Lord will save me, and I will sing praises all the days of my life.

*Surely it was for my benefit that I suffered such anguish.*
*In your love you kept me from the pit of destruction;*
*you have put all my sins behind your back.*
*For the grave cannot praise you, death cannot sing your praise; those who go down to the pit cannot hope for your faithfulness.*
*The living, the living—they praise you, as I am doing today; parents tell their children about your faithfulness.*
*The Lord will save me, and we will sing with stringed instruments all the days of our lives in the temple of the Lord. (Isaiah 38:17-20)*

169

Listen to my cry Lord, for I am in desperate need, rescue me from Lyme disease for it is too strong for me to fight on my own. Set me free from my prison, that I may praise your name. Then people will gather around to listen to my testimony of your goodness to me.

*Listen to my cry, for I am in desperate need;*
*rescue me from those who pursue me, for they are too strong for me.*
*Set me free from my prison, that I may praise your name.*
*Then the righteous will gather about me because of your goodness to me. (Psalm 142:6-7)*

Thank you God that you will provide my every need today and that each day you keep your promises. Thank you that you will deliver me from this pain and suffering and you will honor me for my obedience and faith through it.

*"Sacrifice thank offerings to God, fulfill your vows to the Most High, and call on me in the day of trouble; I will deliver you, and you will honor me." (Psalm 50:14-15)*

Thank you that I can know you Lord and because I put my hope in you, I will not be disappointed.

*Then you will know that I am the Lord; those who hope in me will not be disappointed. (Isaiah 49:23 b)*

God of hope, please fill me will all your joy and peace as I trust in you, so that I may overflow with hope by the power of the Holy Spirit.

*May the God of hope fill you with all joy and peace as you trust in him, so that you may overflow with hope by the power of the Holy Spirit. (Romans 15:13)*

I will be joyful in hope, patient in this affliction, and faithful in prayer.

*Be joyful in hope, patient in affliction, faithful in prayer. (Romans 12:12)*

I know your name and trust in your, for you Lord, will never forsake me because I seek you.

*Those who know your name trust in you, for you, Lord, have never forsaken those who seek you. (Psalm 9:10)*

My God is gracious and righteous and full of compassion. He will protect me when I am brought so low. He will save me. My soul will return to rest for the Lord has been good to me. For you, Lord, have delivered me from death, my eyes from tears, my feet from stumbling, that I may walk before the Lord in the land of the living. I trust in the Lord when I said "I am greatly afflicted."

*The Lord is gracious and righteous; our God is full of compassion.*

*The Lord protects the unwary; when I was brought low, he saved me.*

*Return to your rest, my soul, for the Lord has been good to you.*

*For you, Lord, have delivered me from death, my eyes from tears, my feet from stumbling, that I may walk before the Lord in the land of the living.*

*I trusted in the Lord when I said, "I am greatly afflicted". (Psalm 116:5-10)*

171

God is able to save me completely because I come to him through Jesus who always lives to intercede for me.

*Therefore he is able to save completely those who come to God through him, because he always lives to intercede for them. (Hebrews 7:25)*

The Lord says to me "Do not be afraid or discouraged because of the vast and horrible disease. For the battle is not yours, but God's".

*He said: "Listen, King Jehoshaphat and all who live in Judah and Jerusalem! This is what the Lord says to you: 'Do not be afraid or discouraged because of this vast army. For the battle is not yours, but God's. (2 Chronicles 20:15)*

Thank you Lord, that in this time of grieving what I've lost physically, I will rejoice because no one can take away your joy in me.

*So with you: Now is your time of grief, but I will see you again and you will rejoice, and no one will take away your joy. (John 16:22)*

My flesh and my heart may fail, but God is the strength of my heart and my portion forever.

*My flesh and my heart may fail, but God is the strength of my heart and my portion forever. (Psalm 73:26)*

Give me the Spirit of wisdom and revelation, so that I may know you better. I pray that the eyes of my heart may be enlightened in order that I may know the hope to which You have has called me Lord, the riches of your glorious inheritance in your holy people, and your incomparably great power for me

172

who believes. That power is the same as the mighty strength was exerted when Christ was raised from the dead and seated at his right hand in the heavenly realms, far above all rule and authority, power and dominion, and every name that is invoked, not only in the present age but also in the one to come.

*I have not stopped giving thanks for you, remembering you in my prayers. I keep asking that the God of our Lord Jesus Christ, the glorious Father, may give you the Spirit of wisdom and revelation, so that you may know him better. I pray that the eyes of your heart may be enlightened in order that you may know the hope to which he has called you, the riches of his glorious inheritance in his holy people, and his incomparably great power for us who believe. That power is the same as the mighty strength he exerted when he raised Christ from the dead and seated him at his right hand in the heavenly realms, far above all rule and authority, power and dominion, and every name that is invoked, not only in the present age but also in the one to come. (Ephesians 1:16-21)*

As the years pass through this illness and I grow in age, Lord, do not forsake me. Give me the opportunity to testify of your power and mighty acts in my life to the next generation.

*Even when I am old and gray, do not forsake me, my God, till I declare your power to the next generation, your mighty acts to all who are to come. (Psalm 71:18)*

Thank you Lord, that you will shine on me living in this dark illness and in the shadow of death, and will guide my feet into the path of peace.

*To shine on those living in darkness and in the shadow of death, to guide our feet into the path of peace. (Luke 1:79)*

I keep my eyes always on the Lord. With him at my right hand, I will not be shaken. Therefore my heart is glad and my tongue rejoices; my body also will rest secure, because you will not abandon me to the realm of the dead, nor will you let your faithful one see decay. You make known to me the path of life; you will fill me with joy in your presence, with eternal pleasures at your right hand.

*I keep my eyes always on the Lord. With him at my right hand, I will not be shaken. Therefore my heart is glad and my tongue rejoices; my body also will rest secure, because you will not abandon me to the realm of the dead, nor will you let your faithful one see decay. You make known to me the path of life; you will fill me with joy in your presence, with eternal pleasures at your right hand. (Psalm 16:8-11)*

I love you, Lord, my strength. The Lord is my rock, my fortress and my deliverer;

my God is my rock, in whom I take refuge, my shield and the horn of my salvation, my stronghold. I called to the Lord, who is worthy of praise, and I have been saved from this disease. The cords of death entangled me; the torrents of destruction overwhelmed me. The cords of the grave coiled around me; the snares of death confronted me. In my distress I called to the Lord; I cried to my God for help. From his temple he heard my voice; my cry came before him, into his ears.

*I love you, Lord, my strength. The Lord is my rock, my fortress and my deliverer;*
*my God is my rock, in whom I take refuge, my shield and the horn of my salvation, my stronghold.*
*I called to the Lord, who is worthy of praise, and I have been saved from my enemies. The cords of death entangled me; the*

*torrents of destruction overwhelmed me. The cords of the grave coiled around me; the snares of death confronted me.*

*In my distress I called to the Lord; I cried to my God for help.*

*From his temple he heard my voice; my cry came before him, into his ears.*

*(Psalm 18:1-6)*

I praise you Lord, because you give rest to your people just as you promised and not one good word of yours will fail in all the promises you give.

*Praise be to the Lord, who has given rest to his people Israel just as he promised. Not one word has failed of all the good promises he gave through his servant Moses.*

*(1 Kings 8:56)*

I have this treasure in jars of clay to show that this all-surpassing power is from God and not from me. I am hard pressed on every side, but not crushed; perplexed, but not in despair; persecuted, but not abandoned; struck down, but not destroyed. I always carry around in my body the death of Jesus, so that the life of Jesus may also be revealed in my body. For I, who am alive am always being given over to death for Jesus' sake, so that his life may also be revealed in my mortal body. So then, death is at work in me, but life is at work in every believer.

*But we have this treasure in jars of clay to show that this all-surpassing power is from God and not from us. We are hard pressed on every side, but not crushed; perplexed, but not in despair; persecuted, but not abandoned; struck down, but not destroyed. We always carry around in our body the death of Jesus, so that the life of Jesus may also be revealed in our body.*

175

*For we who are alive are always being given over to death for Jesus' sake, so that his life may also be revealed in our mortal body. So then, death is at work in us, but life is at work in you. (2 Corinthians 4:7-12)*

You are the God of my family and we are your people. Thank you that you promise that I will find favor for surviving this disease and this valley and you will give me rest. Thank you that you love me with an everlasting love and that you draw me with unfailing kindness. You will build me up again, I will be rebuilt. I will go out and dance with the joyful and plant fruit in others' lives.

*"At that time," declares the Lord, "I will be the God of all the families of Israel, and they will be my people." This is what the Lord says:*

*"The people who survive the sword will find favor in the wilderness; I will come to give rest to Israel."*

*The Lord appeared to us in the past, saying: "I have loved you with an everlasting love; I have drawn you with unfailing kindness.*

*I will build you up again, and you, Virgin Israel, will be rebuilt.*

*Again you will take up your timbrels and go out to dance with the joyful.*

*Again you will plant vineyards on the hills of Samaria;*

*the farmers will plant them and enjoy their fruit. (Jeremiah 31:1-5)*

I wait patiently for the Lord; you turned to me and heard my cry. You lifted me out of this illness, and set my feet on a rock and gave me a firm place to stand. You put a new song in my mouth, a hymn of praise to our God. I can tell many of what you have done and they will put their trust in you. Blessed am I, who trusts in the Lord, I will not look elsewhere for my strength. Many, Lord my God, are the wonders you have done, the things you planned for me. None can compare with you; were I to speak and tell of your deeds, they would be too many to declare. Sacrifice and offering you did not desire—but my ears you have opened—burnt offerings and sin offerings you did not require. I desire to do your will, my God; your law is within my heart. I proclaim your saving acts; I will not not seal my lips, Lord. I will speak of your faithfulness and your saving help. I do not conceal your love and your faithfulness. Do not withhold your mercy from me, Lord; may your love and faithfulness always protect me. For troubles in this illness without number surround me; they feel like they could overtake me. My heart fails within me. Be pleased to save me, Lord; come quickly, Lord, to help me. But as for me, I am poor and needy; may the Lord think of me. You are my help and my deliverer; you are my God, do not delay.

*I waited patiently for the Lord; he turned to me and heard my cry.*

*He lifted me out of the slimy pit, out of the mud and mire; he set my feet on a rock*

*and gave me a firm place to stand.*

*He put a new song in my mouth, a hymn of praise to our God. Many will see and fear the Lord and put their trust in him.*

*Blessed is the one who trusts in the Lord, who does not look to the proud, to those who turn aside to false gods.*

*Many, Lord my God, are the wonders you have done, the things you planned for us.*

*None can compare with you; were I to speak and tell of your deeds, they would be too many to declare.*

*Sacrifice and offering you did not desire—but my ears you have opened—burnt offerings and sin offerings you did not require.*

*Then I said, "Here I am, I have come—it is written about me in the scroll.*

*I desire to do your will, my God; your law is within my heart."*

*I proclaim your saving acts in the great assembly; I do not seal my lips, Lord, as you know.*

*I do not hide your righteousness in my heart; I speak of your faithfulness and your saving help. I do not conceal your love and your faithfulness from the great assembly.*

*Do not withhold your mercy from me, Lord; may your love and faithfulness always protect me.*

*For troubles without number surround me; my sins have overtaken me, and I cannot see. They are more than the hairs of my head, and my heart fails within me.*

*Be pleased to save me, Lord; come quickly, Lord, to help me.*

*May all who want to take my life be put to shame and confusion; may all who desire my ruin be turned back in disgrace.*

*May those who say to me, "Aha! Aha!" be appalled at their own shame.*

*But may all who seek you rejoice and be glad in you; may those who long for your saving help always say, "The Lord is great!"*

*But as for me, I am poor and needy; may the Lord think of me. You are my help and my deliverer; you are my God, do not delay. (Psalm 40)*

In my bed and agony, I remember you and think on you throughout the suffering at night. Thank you that you are my help. I sing praises to you in the shadow of your wing in your protection. I will cling to you and your right hand will hold me up.

*On my bed I remember you; I think of you through the watches of the night.*

*Because you are my help, I sing in the shadow of your wings. I cling to you; your right hand upholds me. (Psalm 63:6-8)*

I would have given up if I did not delight in you. I will never forget your promises, for by them you have preserved my life.

*If your law had not been my delight, I would have perished in my affliction.*
*I will never forget your precepts, for by them you have preserved my life.*
*(Psalm 119:92-93)*

Help me Lord to forget the way my life used to be and not dwell in the past. You are doing a new thing in me spiritually, emotionally, and physically. You are making a way for me through this wilderness and wasteland.

*Forget the former things; do not dwell on the past. See, I am doing a new thing!*
*Now it springs up; do you not perceive it? I am making a way in the wilderness and streams in the wasteland. (Isaiah 43:18-19)*

You Lord are the everlasting God, the Creator of the ends of the earth. You will not grow tired or weary, and your understanding I cannot fathom. You will give strength to the me in this weariness and increases the power of the my weak body. Even youths grow tired and weary, and young men stumble and fall; but I will hope in the Lord and you will renew my strength. I will soar on wings like eagles; I will run and not grow weary, I will walk and not be faint.

*Do you not know? Have you not heard? The Lord is the everlasting God, the Creator of the ends of the earth. He will not grow tired or weary, and his understanding no one can fathom.*

*He gives strength to the weary and increases the power of the weak. Even youths grow tired and weary, and young men stumble and fall; but those who hope in the Lord will renew their strength. They will soar on wings like eagles; they will run and not grow weary, they will walk and not be faint. (Isaiah 40:28-31)*

# Postscript

My journey and my valley are not over. Our family's battles continue but we have a winning record. We are chipping away at what Lyme has done in our home.

I am driving, I am reading, and I am writing. Most importantly, I am living. I am living, my eyes focused forward and upward. Trying to see all things He brings each day in light of the character building God is doing in our family.

We are still eating GFCFSF, but all the other sensitivities for the kids are gone. We eat goat's cheese now which is a delicacy in our house and we treasure it. The kids sleep through the night much better, way over half the time. The behavior problems have been severely diminished. My daughter doesn't complain of tummy aches anymore and infrequently launches into prepubescent "tearcapades".

If fact, I can't remember the last time she complained about a tummy ache. Wow. We have come a long way and as I write this, it is a good reminder to be thankful and continue the fight.

I have gained 25 lbs. back but still have about 5 to go and can't seem to put it on no matter how much GF dessert I eat (what a problem huh?). But my pants are no longer duct taped up and I can fit into most of my clothes again. I've even graduated away from the "butt pillow" which I had to use for over a year because I was so thin that it hurt to sit at the kitchen table in our wood chairs without padding.

When we have "regressions" with my son, I claim and remember these things He has accomplished and hold fast to the journey to fight and finish it off.

When I look in the mirror now I see a ton of more gray hairs, but I see life. I see my soul reflecting back a life that was worth fighting for and worth keeping.

My goal for myself and my kids is to live life to the full knowing that each breath is a gift from God. For us to use our talents and experiences to help others find hope and healing. In small measure, I pray for continued strength and for cow's cheese to re-enter our house to be devoured in late night snacks.

My son's goal is to someday eat Papa John's pizza. Maybe someday we will. But until then, I just found out a new pizza place down the street is serving gluten free pizza...

I would encourage each of you to journal this process. Document somehow, via Facebook, blog or writing how you survived and thrived in the valley. Let it be a testimony to others of God's faithfulness and goodness. Use this period in your life to help make His name great. Help other's struggling with Lyme or other debilitating illnesses or physical ailments. Tell Him to let Him use you to help others and to be that testimony. I call it being a Lyme evangelist. This Lyme disease is the most undiagnosed illness in our country. Help others identify and get on the right path. Pray for them. Encourage them.

*Dear Friends, I pray that you may enjoy good health and that all may go well with you, even as your soul is getting along well. (3 John 2) I pray that the Lord will heal all your diseases (Psalm 103:3) and be your strength every morning and be your salvation in your distress. (Isaiah 33:2) I pray that for you who fear His name, the Sun of Righteousness will rise with healing in his wings. And you will go free, leaping with joy like calves let out to pasture. (Malachi 4:2) I pray that your suffering now is nothing compared to the glory God will reveal to you later. (Romans 8:18)*

# Glossary

**Ammonia** - is a compound of nitrogen and hydrogen with the formula NH3 . ammonia is both caustic and hazardous. It is a by product of the die off of Lyme disease and its co-infections.

**Ammonia Toxicity** - has been shown to induce swelling of astrocytes in the brain

**Asperger's** - is an autism spectrum disorder (ASD) that is characterized by significant difficulties in social interaction and nonverbal communication, alongside restricted and repetitive patterns of behavior and interests. It differs from other autism spectrum disorders by its relative preservation of linguistic and cognitive development. Although not required for diagnosis, physical clumsiness and atypical (peculiar, odd) use of language are frequently reported.

**Autism Spectrum Disorder (ASD)-** Autism, Asperger syndrome, pervasive developmental disorder not otherwise specified (PDD-NOS), childhood disintegrative disorder, and Rett syndrome, although usually only the first three conditions are considered part of the autism spectrum. These disorders are typically characterized by social deficits, communication difficulties, stereotyped or repetitive behaviors and interests, and in some cases, cognitive delays.

**Autonomic Nervous System** - is the part of the peripheral nervous system that acts as a control system, functioning largely below the level of consciousness, and controls visceral functions.[1] The ANS affects heart rate,digestion, respiratory rate, salivation, perspiration, pupillary dilation, micturition (urination), and sexual arousal. Most autonomous functions are involuntary but a number of ANS actions can work alongside some degree of conscious control. Everyday examples include breathing, swallowing, and sexual arousal, and in some cases functions such as heart rate.

**Chronic cerebrospinal venous insufficiency (CCSVI or CCVI)** - a term developed by Italian researcher Paolo Zamboni in 2008 to describe compromised flow of blood in the veins draining the central nervous system

**Chronic Lyme Disease** – Having Lyme disease more than 4 weeks (as defined by the CDC) and suffering severe debilitating pain and illness for prolonged period of time.

**Co-infections** – Other pathogens that can be carried with the Lyme spirochete into the body simultaneously that can also cause damage and fatalities. Babesia, Bartonella, Ehrlichia, Colorado Tick Fever, Tick Relapsing Fever, Q Fever, Flavivirus, Rocky Mountain Spotted Fever, West Nile Virus, Tularemia, Micoplasma

**Die Off** – The affect of the body processing the toxic out put from bacteria, viruses, parasites, yeasts, etc in the body. It has been likened to a hangover, some more severe than others.

**Herxheimer-** is a reaction to endotoxins released by the death of harmful organisms within the body. In holistic medicine, it is sometimes referred to as a healing crisis, as it may coincide with recovery from an infectious disease, or a course of detoxification. It resembles bacterial sepsis. A byproduct of the spirochetes causes this reaction. Typically, the death of these bacteria and the associated release of neurotoxins occurs faster than the body can remove the substances. It usually manifests within a few hours of the first dose of any treatment to kill off the spirochete. It manifests as fever, chills, rigor, hypotension,headache, tachycardia, hyperventilation, vasodilation with flushing, myalgia (muscle pain), exacerbation of skin lesions and anxiety.

**Lyme** - an infectious disease carried by ticks caused by bacteria of genus Borrelia

**Lymie** – Any person suffering from Chronic Lyme Disease

**Neurotoxin** – The extrement product of the spirochete in its life cycle. Mass amounts are produced when the spirochete "die off". They are an extensive class of exogenous chemical neurological insults which can adversely affect function in both developing and mature nervous tissue.

**Post Lyme Syndrome** - Most medical experts believe that the lingering symptoms are the result of residual damage to tissues and the immune system that occurred during the infection. The body's "memory" of having chronic lyme disease

**Sepsis** - is a potentially deadly medical condition characterized by a whole-body inflammatory state caused by severe infection. It is caused by the immune system's response to a serious infection, most commonly bacteria, but also fungi, viruses, and parasites in the blood, urinary tract, lungs, skin, or other tissues.

**Spirochete** - bacteria, most of which have long, helically coiled (spiral-shaped) cells. The other most commonly known spirochete is syphilis

# Resources

*Lyme:*
The One Minute Cure – Cavanaugh
The Yeast Connection – Crook
Detoxify or Die – Rogers
Beating Lyme Disease – Jernigan
Everyday Miracles by God's Design – Jernigan
Alkalize or Die - Theodore A. Baroody

*Spiritual:*
31 Days of Praise – Warren and Ruth Meyers
Streams in the Desert – Cowman
Jesus Calling – Sarah Young
Jesus Today – Sarah Young
Circle Maker – Mark Batterson
Drawing the Circle – Mark Batterson

*Uplifting and Encouraging Reading:*
Not a Fan – Kyle Idleman
I Am Second - Doug Bender, Sterrett, McCoy
Beautiful Outlaw – Eldridge
George Mueller – autobiography
Gathering Manna – Sue Fallin
Who is this Man? – John Ortberg
If You Want to Walk on Water You Have to get out of the Boat – John Ortberg
Fearless – Max Lucado
He Still Moves Stones – Max Lucado
The Boy Who Came Back From Heaven – Kevin and Alex Malarkey
Heaven is for Real – Todd Burpo
90 Minutes in Heaven – Don Piper

### *Online:*

https://www.facebook.com/justlivinglikethiswithLYME

http://justlivinglikethiswithlyme.com/

http://pinterest.com/jpfairbairn/just-living-like-this-with-lyme/

http://www.zazzle.com/justlivinglyme

www.lymeresearchalliance.org

Hansa Center for Optimum Health - http://hansacenter.com/

www.mercola.com

http://www.youngliving.com

www.bachflower.com

www.ccsvi.org

Lyme Search Engine, by Google - http://www.tiredoflyme.com/

https://sites.google.com/site/lymediseasemapproject/home

# Chart of Symptoms

*Head, Face, Neck:*
- Headaches/Migraines
- Facial paralysis (like Bell's palsy)
- Tingling of nose, cheek, or face
- Stiff neck
- Sore throat, swollen glands
- Heightened allergic sensitivities
- Twitching of facial/other muscles
- Jaw pain/stiffness (like TMJ)
- Change in smell, taste

*Digestive/excretory System:*
- Upset stomach (nausea, vomiting)
- Irritable bladder
- Unexplained weight loss or gain
- Loss of appetite, anorexia

*Eye, Vision:*
- Double or blurry vision, vision changes
- Wandering or lazy eye
- Conjunctivitis (pink eye)
- Oversensitivity to light
- Eye pain or swelling around eyes
- Floaters/spots in the line of sight
- Red eyes
- Vertigo

*Ears/Hearing:*
- Decreased hearing
- Ringing or buzzing in ears
- Sound sensitivity
- Pain in ears

*Musculoskeletal System:*
- Joint pain, swelling, or stiffness
- Shifting joint pains

- Muscle pain or cramps
- Poor muscle coordination, loss of reflexes
- Loss of muscle tone, muscle weakness

### Respiratory/Circulatory Systems:
- Difficulty breathing. Night sweats or unexplained chills
- Heart palpitations
- Diminished exercise tolerance
- Heart block, murmur
- Chest pain or rib soreness

### Psychiatric Symptoms:
- Mood swings, irritability, agitation
- Depression and anxiety
- Personality changes
- Malaise
- Aggressive behavior / impulsiveness
- Suicidal thoughts (rare cases of suicide)
- Overemotional reactions, crying easily Disturbed sleep: too much, too little, difficulty falling or staying asleep
- Suspiciousness, paranoia, hallucinations
- Feeling as though you are losing your mind
- Obsessive-compulsive behavior
- Bipolar disorder/manic behavior
- Schizophrenic-like state, including hallucinations

### Neurologic System:
- Numbness in body, tingling, pinpricks
- Burning/stabbing sensations in the body
- Burning in feet
- Weakness or paralysis of limbs
- Tremors or unexplained shaking
- Seizures, stroke
- Poor balance, dizziness, difficulty walking
- Increased motion sickness, wooziness
- Lightheadedness, fainting Encephalopathy (cognitive impairment from brain involvement)
- Encephalitis (inflammation of the brain)

- Meningitis (inflammation of the protective membrane around the brain)
- Encephalomyelitis (inflammation of the brain and spinal cord)
- Academic or vocational decline
- Difficulty with multitasking
- Difficulty with organization and planning
- Auditory processing problems
- Word finding problems
- Slowed speed of processing

***Cognitive Symptoms:***
- Dementia
- Forgetfulness, memory loss (short or long term)
- Poor school or work performance
- Attention deficit problems, distractibility
- Confusion, difficulty thinking
- Difficulty with concentration, reading, spelling
- Disorientation: getting or feeling lost

***Skin Problems:***
- Benign tumor-like nodules
- Erethyma Migrans (rash)
- Eczema
- Odd odors or higher perspiration than normal (ammonia)

***General Well-being:***
- Decreased interest in play (children)
- Extreme fatigue, tiredness, exhaustion
- Unexplained fevers (high or low grade)
- Flu-like symptoms (early in the illness)
- Symptoms seem to change, come and go
- Low body temperature
- Other Organ Problems:
- Dysfunction of the thyroid (under or over active thyroid glands)
- Liver inflammation
- Bladder & Kidney problems (including bed wetting)

***Reproduction and Sexuality***
***Females:***
- Unexplained menstrual pain, irregularity
- Reproduction problems, miscarriage, stillbirth, premature birth, neonatal
- Death, congenital Lyme disease
- Extreme PMS symptoms
***Males:***
- Testicular or pelvic pain
***Autoimmune Disorders:***
- Acute Coronary Syndrome
- Fibromyalgia
- Chronic Fatigue Syndrome
- Hashimoto's Hypothyroidism
- Graves' Disease/Hyperthyroidism
- Rheumatoid Arthritis
- Krohns Disease
- Irritable Bowel Syndrome
- Sjogren's Syndrome
- Parkinsons'
- Multiple Sclerosis
- Alzheimer's
- Dimentia
- Lupus
- Depression
- Autism
- ADHD
- Aspergers
- Dyslexia
- Psychological Disorders – Obsessive Compulsive, etc.
- Meniere's
- TMJ
- Celiac
- Addison's Disease
- Diabetes

- Cushing's Disease
- Polycystic Ovary Syndrome
- Restless Leg Syndrome
- Schizophrenia

## About the Author

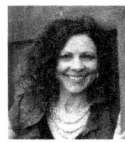 I am a 43 year old married, mother of 2. I discovered I had Lyme disease about 2012, after struggling most of 2011 with severe crashes and health crisis. I apparently had the slow workings of Lyme for over a decade because I gave everything I had to both my kids in the womb. They had been sick since birth and we had no idea what was going on with them. It has been a hard road, one that almost took my life as I hovered under 85 lbs, but it is one that has taught us all great life lessons and strengthened our faith.

As we were climbing out of our Lyme pit in 2013, I realized that God was compelling me to share my journey and give others who suffer a MEASURE OF HOPE.

In my previous life, I was a marketing and communications executive and then a work-from-home and stay-at-home mom. I have now become a PhD in health, healing, living right and all things Lyme. My passion is to see people embrace God's love and faithfulness by providing HOPE for their journey to healing. I love talking about health and healing to anyone who will listen. I adore my kids and how God has used our hardships to grow them into amazing young people with character and perseverance.

softcover book - http://www.amazon.com/author/janicefairbairn
Facebook - https://www.facebook.com/justlivinglikethiswithLYME
Blog - http://justlivinglikethiswithlyme.com/my-blog/
Twitter - https://twitter.com/lymeevangelist
Pintrest - http://www.pinterest.com/jpfairbairn/just-living-like-this-with-lyme/
YouTube - https://www.youtube.com/channel/UCul1VGlVLd6L0IjDwyPCOXg
Tumblr - http://janicelymeevangelist.tumblr.com/
ConnectPal - https://www.connectpal.com/janicefairbairn

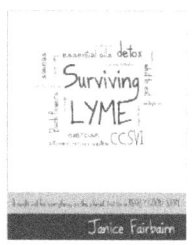

# Surviving LYME

**It might not be everything on the planet, but it's a REALLY GOOD START.**

*Also sold separately or as an ebook.*

- Compact and informative without being overwhelming
- Changing lifestyle choices in small chunks
- Must needs and haves for surviving LYME long term
- Do you want to win the battle or the WAR?

The top survival techniques we used at our house to live through the healing of LYME. Using natural biological methods as a framework, these helpful tips have become part of our family's healing and proactive stance against the Lyme monster.

How Many Different Ways to Heal? Let Me Count Thy Ways.......

Over the dozens of Lymies I've met through the past few years, there are common themed questions and areas that come up the most. I've done my best to document various methods of healing, helping, and surviving LYME disease.

A compilation of different methods used to heal, survive and treat Lyme disease based on our family's experience using non-traditional methods of biological medicine.

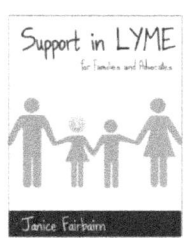

# Support in LYME

## For Families and Advocates

*Also sold separately or as an ebook.*

The LYME Diagnosis is devastating for many people who love a Lymie.

What you need to know to survive a loved one's trial with LYME. How to be a parent of a Lymie, how to be married to a Lymie, or how to be a friend and advocate to one. I cover all the bases on how to live through this with someone fighting to heal and live.

- What to do when you find out your spouse has Lyme
- How to cope with despair and discouragement along the way
- Learn how to be an advocate, fighting for your loved one to succeed
- Glean support and encouragement about how to be the parent of a Lymie child

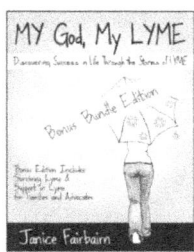

# My God, My LYME

## Discovering Success in Life Through the Storms of LYME - Bonus Bundle

*Also sold separately or as an ebook.*

Prepare for a Radical Battlefield

Be inspired and encouraged by a true journey of faith through LYME. It's an amazing and real life success story. You can't help but be uplifted and gain strength from reading the story of one mom's compelling journey from the brink of death to healing and restoration for herself and her children from LYME.

Giving people the resources and HOPE they need for healing and how to live until they get there. Whether chronically ill with Lyme, already on your path to healing, or if you have conquered the mountain – this is for you.

- Discovering Success in Life out of the Storms of LYME.
- Be Inspired and Encouraged by this Journey of Faith
- Envision and Experience Whole Body Healing
- Prepare for a Radical Battlefield
- Get the Emotional and Spiritual Awakening You Desperately Need

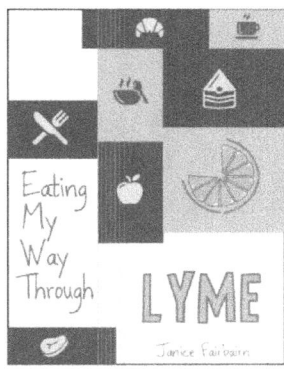

# Don't Eat the Cardboard.

### A Journey Eating My Way Through Lyme.

*Available 2014 ebook.*
*www.selz.com*

# It is so hard to get well and get healthy at the same time.

I know going gluten free or dairy free just makes some of your head's spin. We've been gluten free, soy free and dairy free for almost 10 years now. These are adapted recipes and found recipes and combined recipes I've collected over the years to make our family happy and well fed. You don't have to do the research, you don't have to look for 5 years for a bread recipe that works or a pizza crust recipe your kids will eat – they are all in this collection. I am not a gormet cook, I'm just a mom who wanted to find recipes that worked without too much effort and that my family would enjoy. Your future in gluten free does not have to be bleak – you don't have to eat food that tastes like cardboard the rest of your life!!

*https://justlivinglikethiswithlyme.selz.com/item/548b40d3b798720bbc12c742?mode =edit*

# Coming Soon!

## Available for Pre-Sale on Amazon June 2016

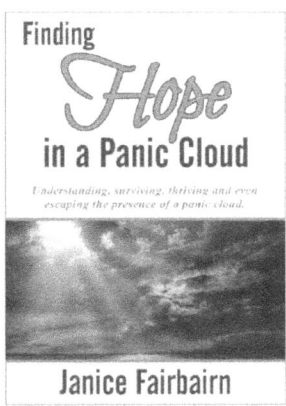

Is the Panic Cloud preventing you from living your life?

Do you feel that if you have faith you shouldn't feel scared or afraid?
Do you feel like if you have God in your life you should never panic?
Do you feel like your faith should keep you from having anxiety attacks in overwhelming situations?

I used to think that I was failing somehow in my faith or that it wasn't strong enough because I felt panic within life's circumstances that were beyond my control. I felt as if I could not breathe at times and that I was destined to live miserable and afraid in a giant Panic Cloud. Sometimes the weight of our trials are a Panic Cloud that envelop and follow you around choking your faith and ability to live. You don't have to feel that way anymore.

There is HOPE.